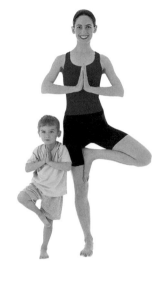

YOGA
FOR YOU
and your child

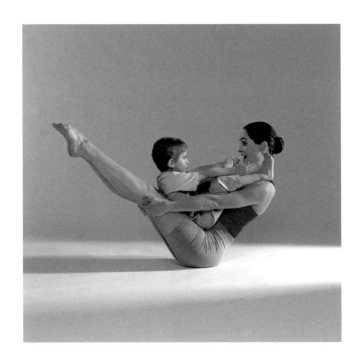

YOGA
FOR YOU
and your child

THE STEP-BY-STEP GUIDE TO
ENJOYING YOGA WITH
CHILDREN OF ALL AGES

MARK SINGLETON

DUNCAN BAIRD PUBLISHERS

LONDON

For the children of the Alice Project.

Yoga for You and Your Child
Mark Singleton

First published in the United Kingdom and Ireland in 2004 by
Duncan Baird Publishers Ltd
Sixth Floor, Castle House
75-76 Wells Street
London W1T 3QH

Conceived, created and designed by Duncan Baird Publishers

Managing editor: Judy Barratt
Editor: Kesta Desmond
Senior designer: Dan Sturges
Commissioned photography: Matthew Ward, Sandra Lousada

British Library Cataloguing-in-Publication Data:
A catalogue record for this book is available from the British Library

10 9 8 7 6 5 4 3 2 1

ISBN: 1-904292-93-3

Typeset in GillSans and Joanna MT
Colour reproduction by Color & Print Gallery
Printed by Imago Singapore

Note on abbreviations:

BCE (Before the Common Era) is the equivalent of BC.
CE (Common Era) is the equivalent of AD.

Publisher's note:
Before following any advice or practice suggested in this book, it is recommended
that you consult your doctor as to its suitability, especially if you or your child suffer
from any health problems or special conditions. The publishers, the author and the
photographers cannot accept responsibility for any injuries or damage incurred as a
result of following the exercises in this book, or of using any of the therapeutic
methods described or mentioned here.

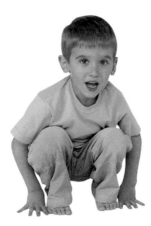

"You are the infinite ocean,
In whom all the things of the world
Rise and fall like waves.

Oh child,
There is nothing to gain,
Nothing to lose,
You are already pure awareness."

Ashtavakra Gita, 15:11–12

contents

foreword

As a small child I went to yoga classes with my mother. We did huge backbends and wobbly handstands; we also roared like lions, hissed like snakes and hummed like bees! There was no performance or competition in these classes, they were just fun. Although I wasn't conscious of it, we were encouraged to be open to the present rather than to strive for a "goal". There was no comparison with others in the class, you just did your own thing.

It was my good fortune that these early experiences of yoga were so positive. I was a deeply unsporty child and this could have resulted in my avoiding any kind of physical activity at all. I loved yoga, though – it gave me a sense of joy in physical being and an appreciation of the power of mental focus without the competitive pressure of team games. The simple practices I learned as a child have stood me in good stead in later life.

My son Milo, now aged four and showing signs of being very sporty, also enjoys yoga. When we practise together, he likes to "correct" me (you can see him doing this on page 31) and he loves animal poses. Despite the fact that I am a yoga teacher, our sessions often end chaotically, with us both rolling on the floor in fits of giggles. We are no more a perfect TV-advertising-style "yoga family" than anyone else! You and your child can do yoga just as well. It can happen right now in your living room, even if you haven't vacuumed the carpet. Just clear a space in the toys and begin!

Yoga provides a special time for both of you – the benefits are not all one way. So often children can remind us to just play and not to try to "learn" or "progress" through conscious effort. Many parents would love to do yoga with their children but are worried about getting it "right". You could not have a better guide than Mark Singleton, an unusually accomplished yoga practitioner and a patient, intuitive teacher. This book is a really comprehensive guide to practising yoga safely and creatively with a child of any age from toddler to teenager. It includes all the essential dos and don'ts, traditional postures that you will recognize from your own yoga classes, as well as lots of imaginative new ideas to encourage exploration and experimentation. Mark's good-humoured and playful teaching style comes across on every page. The gentle and generous quality of his teaching is abundantly clear in his writing.

It is always a challenge for yoga teachers to integrate successfully the philosophical concepts of yoga with the practice of postures and breathing exercises. Perhaps the greatest strength of this book is the seamless melding of philosophy with physical practice. The simple practices shown in this book can form a rock solid foundation from which a child can face the inevitable ups and downs of life. And, at the very least, you will have hours of fun roaring like a lion, hissing like a snake and humming like a bee!

Tara Fraser

introduction

When I was a child I liked to do the lotus pose and walk around the living room on my knees. I was also partial to standing on my head, walking on my hands, arching my back and walking upside-down like a crab. What has stayed with me from those days is the delight that I felt at the unusual things I could do with my body. Back then, of course, I didn't realise that most of these shapes and balances were my own versions of classical yoga postures.

Before I discovered yoga, I had a long interest in education and holistic learning. I taught literature to children in France and the UK, and studied alternative approaches to education. What I discovered was that school children were mostly treated as a head, shoulders, brain and a hand to write with; the rest of them remained hidden behind a desk and a curriculum. When I began to practise yoga I glimpsed a way to help children become body, heart and mind (and all their other aspects) at the same time.

I truly began to understand the potential of yoga for children when I went to teach at the Alice Project, an education experiment in northern India based on the principles of yoga. A high percentage of the children here came from severely disadvantaged backgrounds, and many had been rejected from other schools, either for anti-social behaviour, or because they were too poor to pay the registration fees. After a couple of years at the Alice Project the self-esteem, emotional intelligence, IQ, social skills and academic performance (all closely monitored by the school's psychologist) of almost all the children improved dramatically. In comparison with their peers from neighbouring schools, I found the children extraordinarily friendly, open and aware. I can put this down only to the profoundly healing influence of yoga – the children of the Alice Project not only practised postures, breathing and meditation before class every day, but all of their lessons were interwoven with exercises and meditations adapted from the yoga traditions.

When I returned to the UK, I began teaching yoga in schools and after-school yoga clubs. Once again, I saw the delight and exhilaration of children discovering the infinite potential of their bodies. I noticed again and again how the physical grounding of yoga postures helps to create stability in every other aspect of a child's being. Teaching yoga to kids has shown me how wild – and sometimes destructive – energies can be managed and harnessed creatively. Yoga can also replenish and restore children when they are feeling at a low ebb.

Yoga has given us the tools to help us live in harmony with ourselves and others. If children can learn to use these tools, and apply them to their own lives, then the world will be a brighter and more peaceful place. I wish you all the best on your yoga journey. I hope the games and exercises in this book bring many hours of fun and love, and that you grow together through yoga.

Namaste.

Mark Singleton

how to use this book

You will find in this book everything you need to start practising yoga with your child. Children as young as three and as old as 14 can try the exercises (where appropriate I've included modifications for very young children).

Chapter 1 gives you an overview of yoga and its benefits for children, as well as hints and guidelines for teaching yoga to your child safely and enjoyably. It is a good idea to read this chapter carefully before you go on to the actual postures.

Chapters 2, 3, 4 and 5 are all about *asana*, the physical postures of yoga. For children, this is not only the most relevant and useful aspect of yoga, it's also the most fun. To begin with, focus on the postures in Chapter 2, which warm up the body. Then move on to Chapter 3 which gives you a good grounding in some of the basic classical postures of yoga. Chapters 4 and 5 are full of animal poses, activities, journeys and games – kids love them.

Once you have a grounding in the principles of yoga, use Chapters 2, 3, 4 and 5 as a resource for building your own yoga sessions. Try to stick to the principles of sequencing outlined on page 47. Chapter 6 focuses on *pranayama* (yogic breathwork), meditation and deep relaxation. It will depend on your child as to when you wish to introduce these elements of practice to them (see pages 102 and 109). Chapter 7 includes four sequences that combine many of the postures and techniques that you have learned in other chapters. Chapter 8 addresses how yoga can be used for school. There are exercises based on yoga learning techniques, and advice on how to cope better with stressful exam periods.

However much you learn about yoga from this book, I would always recommend that you and your child go to yoga classes as often as possible. Not only can you both learn things in a class that you can't get from a book, but a class will give you ideas to bring back to your home yoga sessions and keep them fresh and alive.

Yoga for You and Your Child is written for adults, but it can also be read by children. A good idea is to read the book together, so that grown-ups can explain difficult points and children can ask questions. The instructions for the postures and exercises mainly address the child, but adults will need to give occasional help.

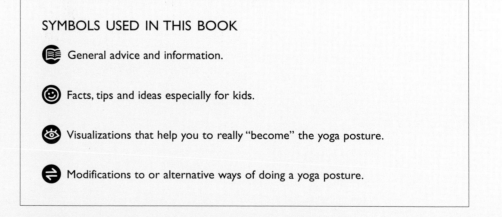

SYMBOLS USED IN THIS BOOK

General advice and information.

Facts, tips and ideas especially for kids.

Visualizations that help you to really "become" the yoga posture.

Modifications to or alternative ways of doing a yoga posture.

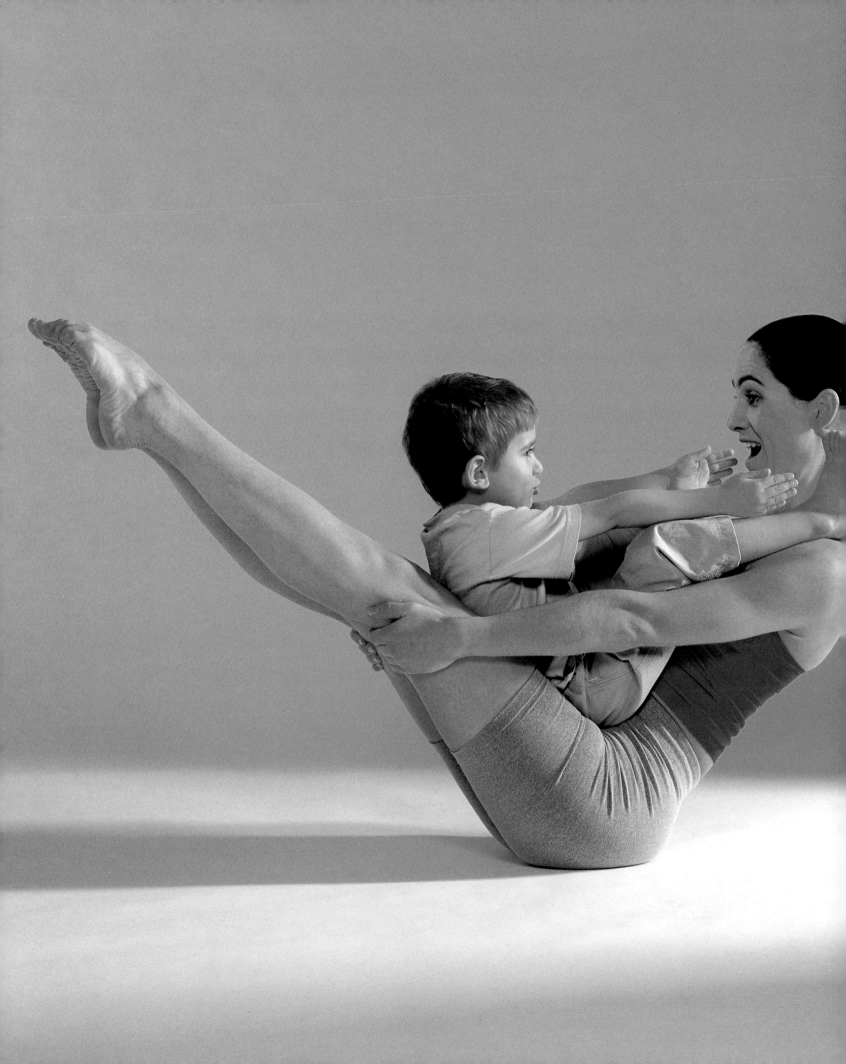

young, open, growing, aware

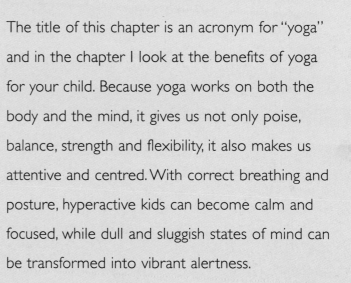

The title of this chapter is an acronym for "yoga" and in the chapter I look at the benefits of yoga for your child. Because yoga works on both the body and the mind, it gives us not only poise, balance, strength and flexibility, it also makes us attentive and centred. With correct breathing and posture, hyperactive kids can become calm and focused, while dull and sluggish states of mind can be transformed into vibrant alertness.

Yoga enhances our awareness of ourselves and the world around us, and this naturally puts us in touch with our spiritual aspect. This is the original purpose of yoga – to open us up to our higher nature, allowing us to celebrate the Divine within.

Children are natural yogis. Good posture, the ability to breathe deeply and an open attitude toward life are things that we are born with. Yoga is the best way to ensure that we don't forget these healthy ways of moving, breathing and being.

growing up fit and strong

In recent years there has been much scientific research into the effects of yoga on children's health. Evidence shows that regular yoga practice can keep children healthy by boosting their immune systems and by keeping their muscles, organs and glands functioning at optimum levels. Yoga also helps children to develop strong, flexible bodies, an excellent sense of balance and coordination, and a feeling of confidence and grace in their movements.

The reason that regular yoga practice is so beneficial in an all-round way is that its postures and breathing techniques are designed to encourage and maintain the flow of *prana* – a basic life-force energy that flows through all living things. When *prana* flows freely, you feel healthy and fit, but when the flow of *prana* is blocked, you become ill.

You can sense *prana* as a tingling or vibrating sensation through your body – it's often possible to feel this during or after yoga. If you encourage your child to be aware of these kinds of sensations during their yoga practice, they will be able to sense when their flow of *prana* is impeded and this will provide them with an excellent early warning of infections such as colds and 'flu.

Standing tall

Yoga also instils good postural habits in children. These days it's common for school-age kids to carry heavy bags or satchels on a daily basis (often over the same shoulder for years), to spend long hours at a school desk and to sit on chairs that encourage slouching and rounding of the lower back (it's interesting that in India there has been a huge rise in the number of back problems since people started sitting on chairs instead of on the floor). Combined with habits such as walking on the outsides of the feet or standing with all your weight on one leg, it's hardly surprising that posture-related problems, most notably backache, are among the most widespread afflictions of modern society.

THE TRADITION OF CHILDREN'S YOGA

In India the traditional way for children to be initiated to yoga was the "thread ceremony" (*upanayavidya* in Sanskrit). Children were taught Greeting the Sun (see pages 43–5), Up and Down the Mountain (see pages 105) and a special prayer to the sun, called the Gyatri Mantra. The sacred thread symbolizes the end of the first stage of childhood and the preparation for adult life. Children went on to study under a *guru* in a special yoga school (a *gurukul*), with each day devoted to the arts of yoga.

The Indian thread ceremony takes place when children reach the age of eight. Here two Gujarati boys prepare to receive the thread.

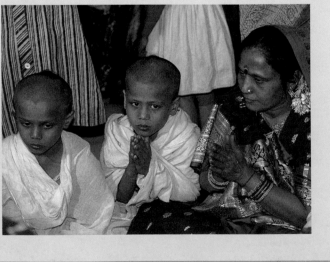

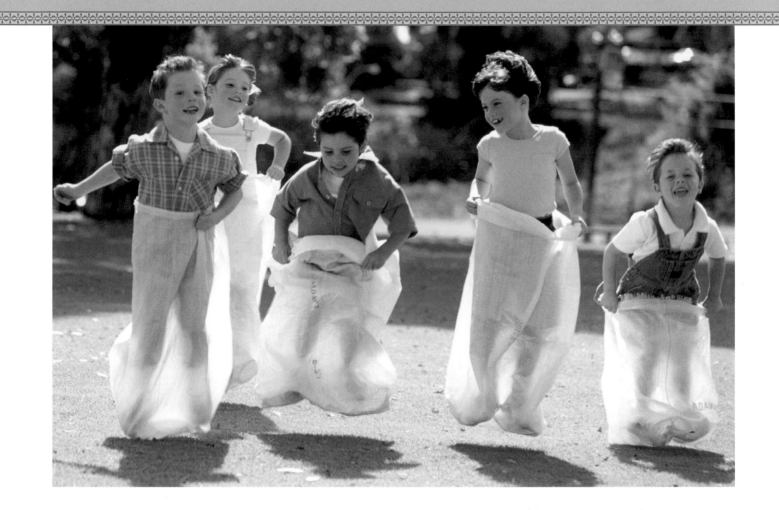

The best way to prevent back problems in later life is to learn good posture at a young age. Practising yoga is an excellent way of doing this – it not only develops a core of strength around the spine and keeps the spine supple and well supplied with blood, but it also teaches children to be aware of the way they carry their bodies, to correct bad habits as they arise and prevent new ones from forming.

Good breathing

Yoga teaches children how to breathe correctly by inhaling slowly and deeply through the nose and drawing the breath right down into their lungs. This type of breathing creates a calm, focused and receptive state of mind (fast, shallow breaths that only get as far as the upper lungs produce a state of agitation that makes it hard to relax or concentrate). Nose

Yoga taps into the energy of the universe and harnesses it for the mind, body and spirit. This is why children who practise yoga regularly are alert and full of vitality, and can immerse themselves wholeheartedly in whatever they do.

breathing, in particular, helps to lengthen the breath and calm us down – it also warms and filters the air before it gets to our lungs. Babies naturally breathe in this way – it is only later on that children pick up the habit of mouth breathing.

If your child suffers from asthma, yogic breathing techniques are especially helpful. Your child will not only learn an awareness of how they breathe – which will help them to correct destructive breathing patterns – but specific techniques can help them to strengthen their respiratory and immune systems and to cope better in the event of an attack.

A PHILOSOPHY FOR LIFE

In the West yoga is sometimes seen simply as a form of exercise. But yoga is actually an ancient spiritual discipline that is designed to prepare the mind and the heart for the Divine. The first person to write down a systematic yoga doctrine was Patanjali between 200BCE and 200CE. In the *Yoga Sutras*, Patanjali said that there are eight aspects, or "limbs", of yoga and that if a person practised each limb with energy, they would eventually reach a state of complete mental and physical wellbeing. Ultimately, they would attain the final goal of yoga, which is union with the eternal aspect of themselves.

The eight limbs, as set out by Patanjali, are as follows:
1. Learning to live in harmony with others (*yama*).
2. Keeping our body, mind and spirit in health and happiness (*niyama*).
3. Practising physical postures to make the body strong (*asana*).
4. Breathing properly in order to manage energy (*pranayama*).
5. Gathering our mental forces into ourselves (*pratyahara*).
6. Focusing our entire attention on a given object (*dharana*).
7. Resting in effortless meditation (*dhyana*).
8. Becoming one with the Infinite (*samadhi*).

Patanjali's eight limbs of yoga work on every aspect of our life: social, behavioural, ethical, moral, physical, emotional, mental and spiritual – areas of life that are often ignored by conventional education. A fully rounded yoga practice that includes posture (see chapters 2–5 and Chapter 7), breathing and meditation (see Chapters 6 and 8) can create balanced, whole and creative children. It can endow both us and our children with psychological health, physical strength and emotional literacy. Above all, it can teach us to have compassion for our fellow human beings.

Through practising yoga children are able to discover a quiet space inside themselves. Eventually, feeling calm and centred becomes a vital component of their identity.

As the incidence of asthma increases (in Australia it is estimated that one in eight children has asthma) and controversy grows about the safety of conventional drug treatments, parents are turning more and more to natural methods of managing the condition.

A calm nervous system

Calming down the nervous system is another critically important role for yoga in children's health. We often, unwittingly, subject children to sensory overload from TV, video games and electronic toys, stress from a hectic, fast-paced lifestyle, and inadequate nutrition from convenience and processed food. The net result is kids who are chronically over-stimulated and who lack the ability to concentrate for sustained periods of time. Behavioural disorders such as attention deficit disorder (ADD) or attention deficit hyper-activity disorder (ADHD) are extreme examples of this.

By working with breath and movement, yoga can slow down a child's heart and breathing rate and strengthen the central nervous system. This has a profoundly calming influence on a child's mental and emotional states. Once children have learned how to be still and quiet, they come to enjoy this feeling and to seek it out for themselves. On a practical level, if your child is prone to tantrums, clumsiness, poor memory or antisocial behaviour, you will find that regular yoga practice can gradually help with these problems.

Learning the theory and practice of yoga is part of daily life in some Indian schools. Here a girl demonstrates Building a Bridge (see pages 84–5) to a group of kindergarten children.

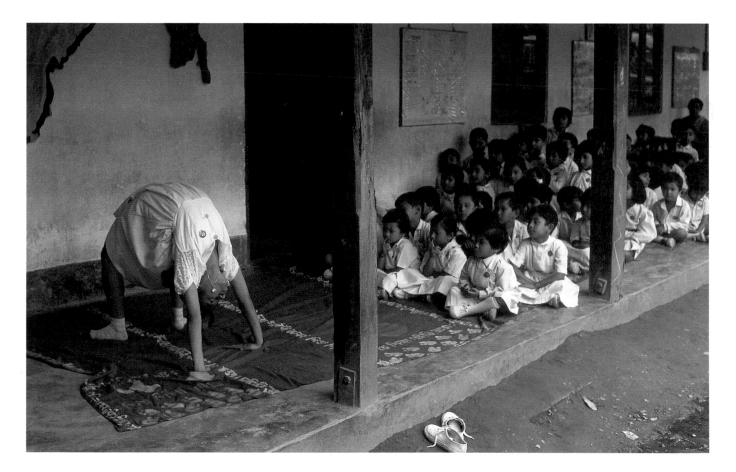

building confidence and focus

In yoga there are no rewards and no punishments, no winners and no losers, no best and no worst. The reward of yoga comes simply from the practice itself. Children love this kind of approach. When they realise that they don't have to compete or perform they start to feel free to express themselves without fear of judgment or criticism. This freedom helps children to develop a sense of confidence and self-esteem that stays with them into adulthood.

The inner confidence that yoga brings is an excellent antidote to the pressure to succeed that children can experience at school. From a very early age, many children learn that to be seen as successful they must strive to be better than their peers. They must get better grades, pass more exams and be "top of the class".

This kind of intense competition makes children hypersensitive to praise and criticism. If they do well at school, they become self-congratulating; if they do less well, they become discouraged and may start to see themselves as failures. Competition inevitably creates an unstable sense of self-esteem – even those children who shine academically can feel that their self-worth rests on their school performance rather than something that is deeper, more enduring and personal.

In contrast, yoga advocates a non-competitive approach to life. Yogic philosophy says that, instead of comparing ourselves with others, we should focus impartially on whatever task we tackle. In the *Bhagavad Gita* (one of the most important ancient texts on yoga written around the 6th century BCE), it says that focusing on the results of our actions leads

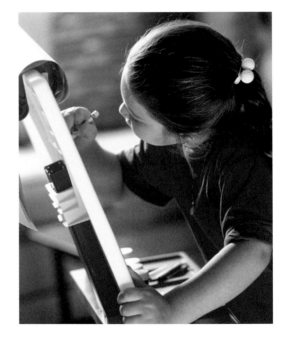

Encouraging your child to express themselves in whatever way comes naturally to them is part of yoga. Children often find it easier to paint or draw their emotions than to express them in words.

to ignorance, whereas working to the best of one's abilities, without anxiety about success or failure, leads to wisdom.

This is why practising yoga in a non-competitive spirit at home with your child can create a wonderful respite from the performance pressure they experience in their daily lives. It's my experience that once kids stop worrying about achievements and results, they begin to enjoy what they are doing in and for itself. And, as a consequence, the quality of their life and work improves.

A place of acceptance

Yoga is about listening to and releasing emotions. Encourage your child to bring issues that are preoccupying or worrying them to your yoga sessions. Listen impartially and without judgment. Your child should feel that they can say anything they want to without fear of blame, anger or criticism. Even if they express negative emotions, they need to know that they can rely upon your ongoing love, acceptance and support.

You can use crayons, pencils or paint to give your child an expressive outlet for difficult or strong emotions. Let them draw or paint how they feel, so that they can discover what colour, shape and size their emotions are. This will help them to enter into a more conscious and sensitive relationship with their inner life.

Another useful exercise is to write down any issues or questions that are troubling you or your child at the beginning of your yoga session. You then put them to one side until the end of the session. The benefits of this are twofold. First, it frees up your attention for the yoga session itself. Second, yoga can often produce the answers you need by allowing you to access the deeper levels of your consciousness. Another good exercise to try if you or your child are feeling upset or anxious is Guardian Angel on page 115.

Changing your mood

Yoga can teach you how to carry your body in a positive way and this has a profound effect on your mood and sense of self-esteem. When people are sad or lacking in confidence they round their shoulders and look down. Angry people stick their chin out and clench their teeth and fists. People who feel happy and confident stand tall with their chest and shoulders open.

Yoga gives children first hand experience of the reciprocal relationship between posture and mood. Through yoga they learn how manipulating posture can create a positive state of mind and counteract a negative one (this is partly why yoga has been so effective in the treatment of problems such as depression and aggression). When you do yoga with your child, get them to explore how different postures make them feel. For example, backbends, such as Building a Bridge (see pages 84–5) and Snake (see page 70) open the heart and make us feel bright and alive. Forward bends, such as Sitting Sandwich (see page 54) and Little Butterfly (see page 72) are soothing and make us feel calm and rested.

Developing mindfulness

Regular yoga practice teaches you to become mindful – this is the ability to immerse yourself completely in the moment without becoming distracted. It means that you are

---

AVOIDING COMPETITION

The best way to discourage competition and ambition in yoga at home is to make your sessions as fun as possible. Make sure that your child is safe and won't hurt or damage themselves, but beyond this, concentrate on creating a sense of freedom and enjoyment.

- Make it clear to your child that not being able to do a posture is nothing to be disheartened or frustrated about and it doesn't affect the way you feel about them. Equally, getting a yoga posture "right" doesn't make your child better than anyone else.
- Avoid making comparisons. Don't compare today's yoga practice with yesterday's – every day is a fresh start. And, if you do yoga with more than one child, never compare their abilities.
- Don't strive to achieve the difficult poses. Take the attitude that yoga is a dance rather than a race.

---

completely at one with whatever you are doing. Mindfulness is the quality that distinguishes a yoga practice from most other kinds of exercise.

Children benefit greatly from mindfulness – their powers of concentration improve and they develop greater awareness of themselves and their surroundings. Instead of being scattered they become focused and attentive.

You can encourage your child to become mindful during yoga practice by getting them to move slowly and to think about how different postures and breathing techniques make them feel. You can also lead by example – do your yoga practice slowly and mindfully and your child will copy you. Children are natural mimics and watching an adult who is absorbed in their yoga practice is infinitely more inspiring than being told to "pay attention".

your inner yoga space

If you have done yoga before, you have probably experienced that deep sense of peace and stillness that sometimes comes during and after your practice. This is your inner "yoga space". Everyone has it inside them and it always exists, even when you are not aware of it. In this space there is no suffering and nothing to fear. Some people say that it is our Divine Nature, our true home or "who we really are"; others call it the Spirit, the Soul or the Self. It is what connects us to everything else in the universe.

From the moment we are born to the moment we die, we are always changing. Our bodies grow, develop, reach maturity and then gradually become old; our moods, attitudes, beliefs and tastes are perpetually shifting so that we are never exactly the same person that we were last year or even last month. The world around us is also evolving all the time. Yet, in the midst of all this flux, our inner yoga space is the one thing that stays constant and unchanging.

Yoga can help us to connect with and draw strength from this peaceful and unchanging part of ourselves. The word "yoga" means to "join together", and its practices are designed to teach us how to join our "little" or everyday selves with this "bigger" part of ourselves.

The concept of "little self" and "big self" is a useful one to teach to children. Once they have sensed their big self through yoga, they know that, whatever happens in life, they

The waves and the ocean are a good metaphor for the "little self" and the "big self" within us. When we look at the sea we may see only the waves that disrupt the ocean's surface. Likewise, when we look at ourselves, we may see only the "surface-self" of our personality.

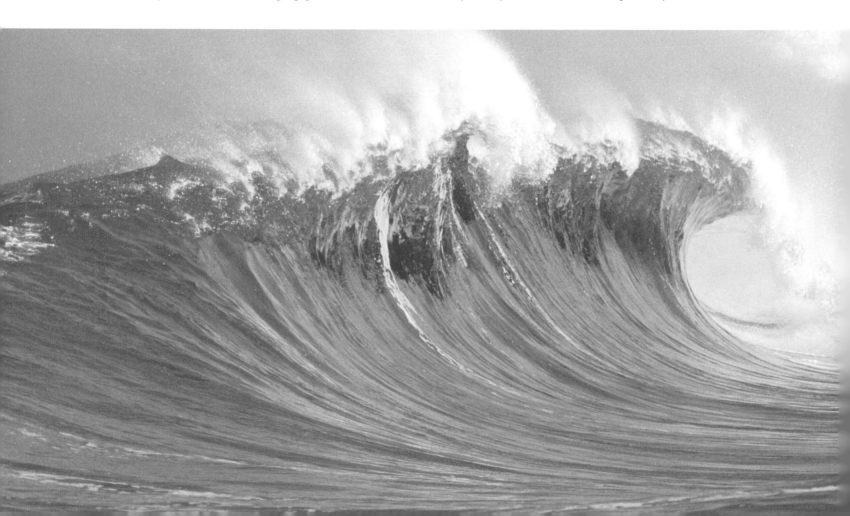

have a safe place to which they can return. As you embark on your yoga journey, your big self will become increasingly familiar. Children especially get to recognize it quickly.

Interconnectedness

Once you are able to access your inner yoga space or "big self" the realization often follows that you are connected to everything else in the universe – that you are part of the same fabric. A good way to explain this idea is to think about the ocean and the waves. Although a wave can seem separate from the ocean in that it has its own shape, direction and momentum, this is in fact an illusion. Wave and ocean are made of the same matter (water) and the wave cannot exist without the support of the ocean all around it. Most importantly, the wave only lasts a minute or two before it disappears back into the ocean. In other words, what we call "big self" and "little self" or "ocean and wave", are actually the same thing. It's only our perception that takes our little self for the whole, and forgets about the big self that we come from. The goal of yoga is to realise this.

Once we stop believing in our separateness from other people and the world around us and begin to believe in our interconnectedness, we become much more selfless and compassionate. If children grow up believing that they are part of a greater whole, they will naturally have respect for other people and the world in which they live.

The tool that you use to contact your big self is mindfulness (see page 21). This is why many of the practices in this book encourage you and your child to find out how you are feeling and what your body and mind are saying to you. Tuning into yourself like this gives you great clarity. Instead of being swamped by your moods and emotions, you learn to see them for what they are: mere waves on a vast ocean.

The desire dragon

One issue that all parents face is how to deal with demands that they can't or don't want to meet. When children decide that they must have something – whether it's a toy, a bar of

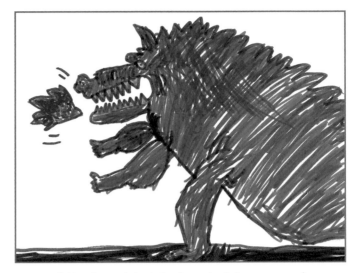

Let your child understand the desire dragon in their own way – for example, by drawing it or imitating its fiery breath. When children are able to sense that the desire dragon is just a superficial part of a much bigger self they will find it much easier to let go of their desires and cravings.

chocolate or a pair of trainers – it can be difficult to persuade them otherwise. We often end up saying an angry "no" or giving in, neither of which is particularly useful.

The persistent feeling of wanting something is what I call the "desire dragon". It makes us feel bad, and the more intense the craving, the more dominated and distracted by it we are. And, if we finally get what we want, it only satisfies us briefly. Before long, we start to desire the next thing that we think will make us happy. This is how many of us spend our whole lives – as slaves to the desire dragon – grasping for external rewards and material possessions, forgetting that true contentment comes from within. If you can help your child to understand this, you will be teaching them one of the deepest truths of life. Many of the most important teachings of yoga and Buddhism are based on the understanding that satisfaction comes from *being* rather than from *having*.

Describe the desire dragon to your child in language that they understand. By contacting your inner yoga space you and your child will come to understand the desire dragon, and learn to distinguish between cravings and real needs.

getting started

The most important thing when you start to practise yoga at home is that you allow your child to be as creative and imaginative as possible. Always be prepared to deviate from a pre-arranged sequence of postures. Let your child suggest ideas, dress up, make noises and even invent their own postures, games and adventures. Encourage them really to *become* the postures, rather than just doing them.

How old?

Children can begin to practise yoga as early as three or four years old. However, every child is different and you are the best judge of when your child is receptive to yoga. Bear in mind that children of three and four will have less developed motor skills than their older counterparts, and their sense of balance will be less good. Postures that require a combination of strength, balance and co-ordination such as Half Moon (see page 51) or Greeting the Sun (see pages 44–5) may be too challenging, so concentrate on easier poses, such as Little Butterfly (see page 72) or Sitting Sandwich (see page 54). Young children respond to yoga best when it is presented as purposeful play rather than as formal practice.

Once you have built up a knowledge of the postures in this book you will know what is right for your child. As your child gets older, gradually introduce a greater variety of postures – and if a posture doesn't seem to be working, just stop doing it and re-introduce it a few weeks or months later.

Your practice space

It doesn't matter in which room of your house you practise yoga as long as it is safe. Always move furniture out of the way, get rid of any sharp corners, and put blankets or cushions over any hard surfaces or angles. Beyond this, try to make the room as comfortable and child-friendly as possible. You may like to build a little "yoga shrine" as a focal point for the room. You and your child can arrange objects that represent peace and beauty for you both – these could be natural objects such as flowers, pebbles or shells, photographs of people or places, or images or icons from your own religious or spiritual tradition.

You may also like to have a CD-player in your yoga room so that you can play relaxing or inspiring music. On a practical level, you should put blankets or a couple of "sticky" yoga mats on the floor to provide a firm, comfortable surface as you do the postures.

How often?

When you are just starting yoga it's better not to have a strict timetable that you feel obliged to follow. Do yoga when it feels right and when you and your child are both feeling really keen. This way you come to the practice full of enthusiasm and interest. Above all, never make your child do yoga if they don't feel like it. Encourage them to find their own ways of imposing routine and discipline.

Later, once the yoga bug has taken hold, you can work out a regular practice time with your child – say, two or three (or more, if you're enthusiastic) times a week before or after school, at the same hour. It is through regular practice that you derive the greatest physical and emotional benefits from yoga. And kids thrive on regularity and routine.

How long?

When you are just starting yoga, keep your sessions short – around five to ten minutes can be plenty. Later, when you and your child are accustomed to doing yoga together, you can lengthen the time of the session. For example, some of the sequences in Chapter 7 last up to 45 minutes.

If you're in any doubt about how long your yoga session should last, let your child guide you. Start to wind down the session once your child shows signs of boredom or fatigue. This will prevent yoga from becoming a chore.

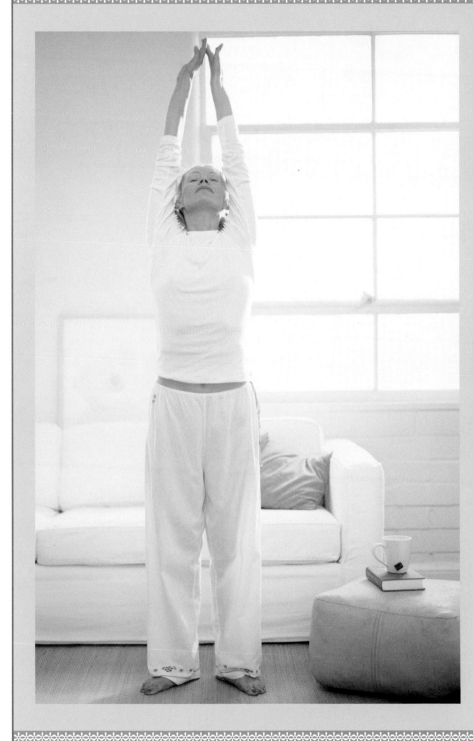

YOUR YOGA
AND THEIR YOGA

Before you start practising yoga with your child it's essential that you gain some personal and practical experience of yoga by going to classes yourself. This will help you to understand the postures and breathing techniques. It will also give you a "feeling" for yoga, which you will then naturally bring home to the sessions that you share with your child.

It's also important that you make a distinction between the yoga that you do for yourself and the yoga that you do with your child. Apart from the fact that children need an individually-tailored practice (young children don't possess the attention span or the physiology to hold postures for the same length of time as an adult), you will benefit from doing your own dedicated yoga sessions. They will help you to build an inner reserve of strength and peace that provides an antidote to stress. Remember that when you do yoga, you become a child yourself: receptive, alert and learning.

Once you have learned some of the basics of yoga in a class you should start regular self-practice at home. The valuable thing about the yoga that you do by and for yourself is that it gives you the chance to relinquish the role of parent and enjoy some solitary self-exploration.

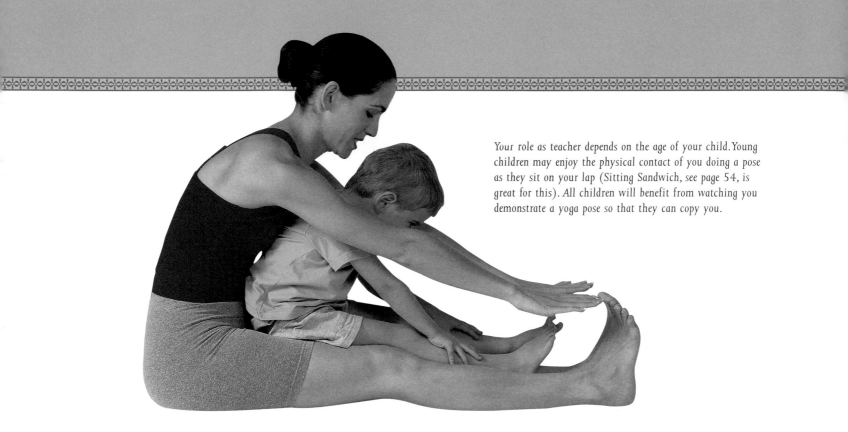

Your role as teacher depends on the age of your child. Young children may enjoy the physical contact of you doing a pose as they sit on your lap (Sitting Sandwich, see page 54, is great for this). All children will benefit from watching you demonstrate a yoga pose so that they can copy you.

Your role as teacher

When you first start to practise yoga with your child you will need to take on a fairly active teaching role. Start by looking at the postures in this book and trying them out for yourself so that you understand each one from the inside. Then demonstrate the postures to your child – once they have a "visual" of a posture, they will be much more prepared to try it out themselves.

Talk your child through each stage of a posture, showing them how to get into and out of it. If they are at the stage of synchronizing breath and movement (see page 102), tell them when to breathe in and out. Gently correct any mistakes or misunderstandings and give your child heaps of praise and encouragement. Try going over the postures at the end of your session by looking at the photographs in this book and reminding yourselves of the names. This will help your child to remember them next time. Don't bother doing this if it feels like a chore though.

Later, when you and your child are familiar with the postures, you can adopt the role of facilitator rather than teacher. Do the poses alongside your child and offer assistance or guidance when it is needed.

Always make sure your child's yoga practice is a safe one. Children's joints are delicate and can be easily damaged. If your child tells you that a certain movement or posture hurts, bring them out of it immediately and try to find the source of the pain. Are they doing the posture incorrectly or pushing too hard? If you can't rectify the problem, seek the advice of an experienced children's yoga teacher.

A good way to avoid placing stress on the joints is to practise each posture dynamically – this means going in and out of the posture several times, rather than holding it for a prolonged period.

Laugh at failures

Try to find the right mixture of challenge and support in your yoga practice, so that your child doesn't feel threatened or bored. If you're doing something new or difficult, make it into an entertaining game, where a spectacular "failure" is just as fun and exciting as getting a posture "right". This teaches children never to be afraid to do something for fear of failure. Approach the journey of yoga with the attitude that what matters is how much fun you have along the way, not how quickly you travel.

Tailor your practice

Like adults, children have days when they feel lively and energetic and days when they feel more quiet and introspective. Always try to tailor your yoga session to your child's mood. Have plenty of ideas up your sleeve and keep things varied and fun for the energetic days. Likewise, keep things simple and peaceful for the quiet days. (I have designed some of the sequences in Chapter 7 for different moods and energy levels.) If you choose to play music during your yoga sessions it's a good idea to reserve some CDs for especially active or especially quiet occasions.

Whatever type of practice you do, always try to end each session by doing some calming and focusing exercises (see Chapter 6), and lying down in *Shavasana* (see page 32). This is important in order to assimilate all of the physical, emotional and spiritual benefits of doing yoga.

Respect your child's moods and energy levels by adapting your yoga practice as necessary or, if they are old enough, letting them lead the session themselves. If your child is in a quiet mood just practise a short series of sitting or lying postures.

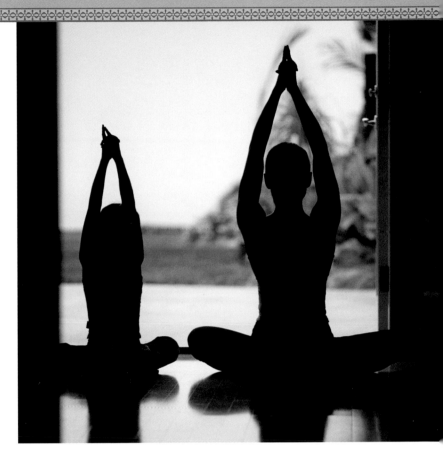

JUST BEFORE YOU START...

Here are some practical pointers for immediately before you and your child begin a yoga session.

- Tell everyone else in your house that you are about to start yoga and that they shouldn't disturb you. Alternatively, you could invite them to join in.
- Turn off any phones, computers or other electronic distractions or get someone else to field any messages.
- Leave your day-to-day chores and duties at the yoga room door. Let this time be completely free from worries about the past or the future. You can act this out by throwing all of

your worries into a bin, and leaving it outside the door. Then be fully present in the moment with your child.
- Make sure that you don't have a full stomach. The ideal time to practise yoga is before breakfast when your stomach is empty. If you are practising in the afternoon or evening, try to leave at least a couple of hours between your last meal and the yoga session.
- If your child is feeling hungry before a practice, give them a glass of milk or a few grapes to boost their blood sugar levels and ward off hunger. However, you will usually find that any hunger pangs disappear once you start your session.

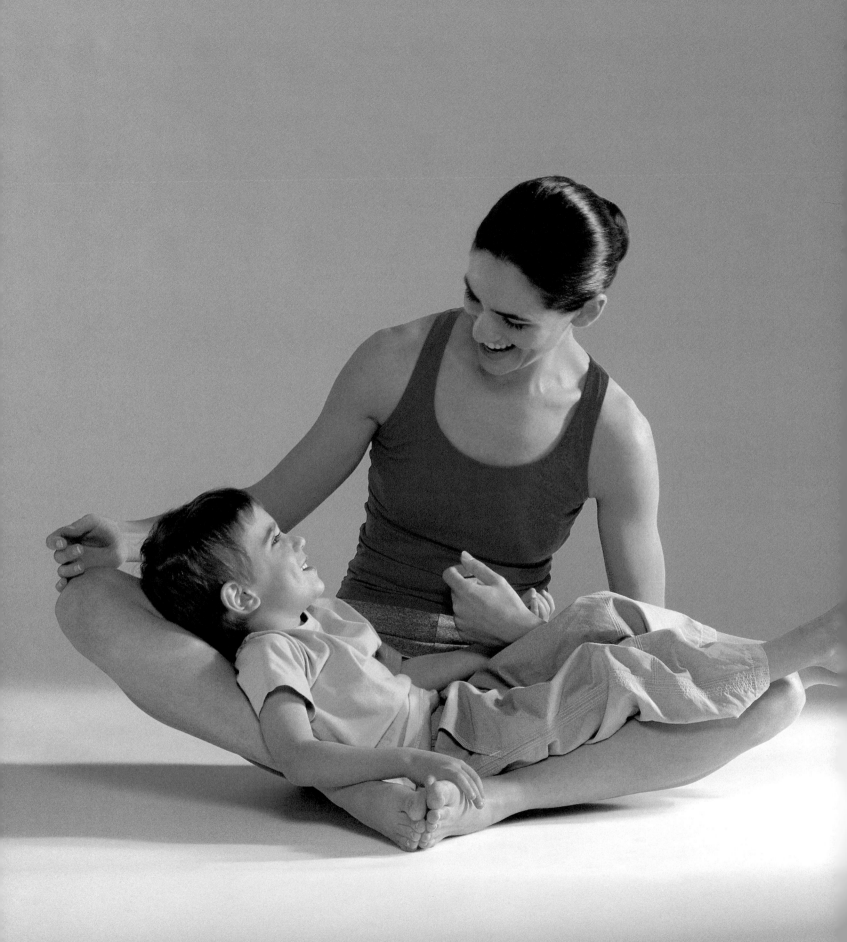

waking up and warming up

The postures in this chapter will warm up your body and loosen your limbs and joints before your main yoga session. You can also treat the postures as a yoga practice in their own right. The Greeting the Sun sequence on pages 44–5 is a particularly good self-contained yoga practice.

The chapter starts by explaining how to tune into your physical and mental state and find a place of calm. Then there are six lying postures to restore energy and prepare you gently for your yoga session – useful after a long day at work or school. The next six standing postures are more vigorous and dynamic. They'll get your joints and muscles oiled and moving, and wake you up.

You can practise the lying and standing postures individually or as a continuous sequence. As you get used to doing the postures with your child, you'll find that you are able to choose exactly the right poses to match your mood and energy levels.

checking in

Sitting quietly with your child for two or three minutes and focusing on your body and your environment helps to prepare you for the yoga session that you are about to begin. Children especially can build incredible self-awareness through this simple practice. It also lets you and your child connect with each other in a spirit of love and understanding.

How much emphasis you put on Checking In depends on the age and disposition of your child. If your child is very young, easily distracted or you're just starting yoga, keep it short – a minute can be plenty. On some days, you may even want to go straight into posture practice.

1 Sit cross-legged on the floor on the edge of a folded blanket or a cushion (if you find it difficult to sit on the floor, sit on a chair). You should be comfortable, relaxed and alert. Get your child to sit opposite you and hold your hands. If they are very young, they can sit on your lap. Gently close your eyes and become as still as a rock. Your child can either keep their eyes open or close them.

2 Encourage your child to focus on the sounds that they can hear. Guide their awareness with these questions: "Which sounds are coming from inside the room? Which sounds are coming from outside? Which sounds are coming from your own body? Can you hear your breath or your heart?" Now get them to think about bodily sensations such as touch and temperature. Ask them: "Which parts of your body are touching the floor? How does it feel to hold my hands? Do you feel hot or cold? Touch your legs, your back, your front, your neck and head – how do they feel? How does your face feel?"

expressing emotion

The start of a yoga session is a good time for you and your child to tune into your moods and emotions. Children often find it easier to express emotions physically rather than in words, and the following exercises can help them to do this.

📖 Try not to speak during the exercises – wait until afterward to talk about what you were feeling and thinking. And always keep the exercises light and humorous.

📖 Make step 2 into a game in which your child moulds you into a range of shapes and you have to guess the emotion each time.

I Encourage your child to adopt the posture or shape that best fits how they are feeling. This can be any shape at all. Encourage them to use their hands and face and to be as expressive as possible. Ask them if there is any noise that they want to make to accompany the shape.

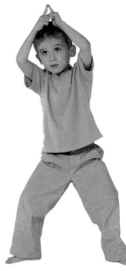

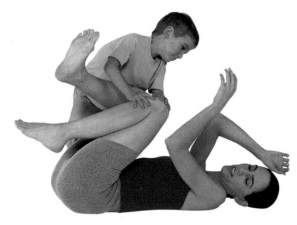

2 Tell your child that you are a piece of plasticine and that they have to mould you into the shape that best represents their mood. Encourage them to get the details just right, even down to the position of your fingers, eyebrows and mouth. Now ask your child to mirror the posture back to you.

FINDING A PLACE OF CALM

A traditional way to start a yoga practice is to chant the sacred syllable "OM" – this represents the Divine Nature within us all and is said to be the original sound of the universe. Chanting OM focuses your attention, makes your mind calm and receptive and signals the start of your special yoga time. Take a deep breath in and make an "o" shape with your mouth. Then let out a long "o" sound followed by a short "mmmm" sound. For example, if your "o" lasts five seconds, your "mmmm" should last one second. Repeat this three times. Children quickly learn to love hearing and feeling the syllable vibrating through their bodies.

Another good way to start your yoga practice in a peaceful and positive frame of mind is to say a prayer or an "aspiration". This can be whatever you want it to be – anything from a prayer from your own religious tradition to a positive statement of who you want to become. You might simply say, "Today I will smile at everything that happens to me, good or bad."

shavasana sandwich

Shavasana involves lying quietly in a mindful state. Although it looks easy, it's quite difficult to do properly, because we're not used to staying still for long. It is a good pose to restore energy at the beginning and the end of your yoga session – it can make you feel as refreshed and rested as deep sleep. In *Shavasana* Sandwich, you and your child lie together, listening to the beating of your heart and feeling the rise and fall of your chest and belly as you breathe.

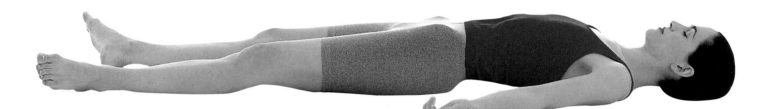

Lie down on your back, with your feet a bit wider than hip-distance apart and falling out to the sides. Check that your body is symmetrical and your head is straight. Move your arms a little way from your body with your palms facing up. This is *Shavasana*.

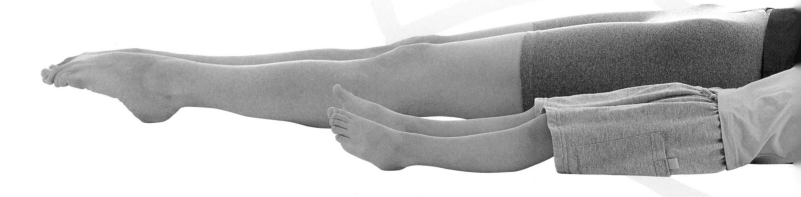

If your child is too big or heavy to lie on top of you, they can lie on the floor at a right angle to you with their head on your abdomen. Their head is gently rocked by the wave-like movement of your belly as you breathe. This will lull them into a deeply relaxed state. Release this position slowly, as described in step 3.

2 Lift your child or get them to climb on top of you. Let them find a comfortable lying position on their front with one ear against your chest so that they can hear your heart. Both close your eyes. Encourage your child to follow the slow, steady rise and fall of your chest and belly as you breathe. Become as quiet and relaxed as possible, bathing in a sense of stillness and warmth. This is *Shavasana* Sandwich. If you are cold, put a blanket over you both.

3 When you feel rested and replenished, slowly separate yourselves and lie side by side. Take your arms above your heads and stretch your entire body from your fingertips down to your toes.

rocking the boat and dead bug

Rocking the Boat gently massages your spine and the large muscles on either side of it. The posture stretches and kneads your vertebrae and discs and stimulates your entire nervous system – this is revitalizing when you feel stiff or tired. The second posture, Dead Bug, activates your hip joints and releases accumulated tension and emotion – we store a lot of stress, fatigue and anxiety in our hips.

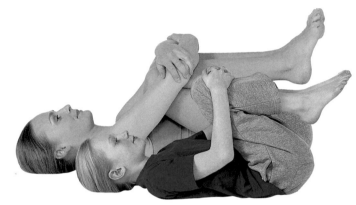

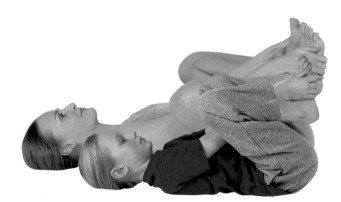

1 Lie on your back and draw your knees toward your chest – wrap your arms around your knees and draw them closer. Rock gently from side to side between 10 and 20 times. Keep your head on the floor. Enjoy your back being massaged by the floor. This is Rocking the Boat.

👁 Pretend that you are lying in a boat that is rocking gently on a blue sea. Imagine that the sun's rays are warming your face.

2 Release your knees and let them come apart. Reach between your knees with your hands and take hold of the outside edges of your feet. Keep your head on the floor with your neck relaxed.

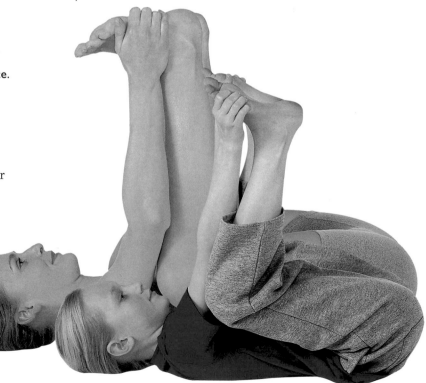

3 Move your feet so that the soles face the ceiling. Gently pull down on your feet so that your knees move toward the floor on either side of your body. Your shins should be vertical and your lower back pressed against the floor. This is Dead Bug. Relax into the pose and make a buzzing noise on each exhalation – make the buzzing last as long as you can.

📖 The "buzzing breath" helps you to become conscious of your breath and naturally lengthens your exhalation which has enormous benefits (see page 107) for both your body and mind.

rolling twist

This lying twist stimulates your whole spine, expelling stagnant blood and letting fresh blood flood in. It keeps your digestive system working efficiently and is sometimes recommended as a cure for constipation. You can go straight into this posture from Dead Bug (see opposite).

1 From Dead Bug, let go of your feet and bring your knees together as close to your chest as you can. Stretch your arms out to the sides with your palms facing up.

2 As you breathe out, bring your knees down toward the floor on the right side of your body. Make sure that your left shoulder doesn't come off the floor. Look toward your left hand. As you breathe in, bring your knees back to the centre. As you breathe out, move your knees over to the left, making sure that your right shoulder doesn't come off the floor. Look toward your right hand. Do the whole movement 5 to 8 times, then stretch out your legs and relax.

dynamic easy bridge

This backbending posture is wonderful for waking up your spine and energizing you. It stretches the front of your body and opens out your chest and shoulders, helping you to breathe more fully. It also strengthens the muscles in your legs and buttocks.

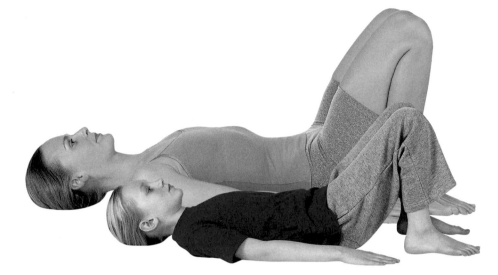

1 Lie down on your back. Bend your knees and bring your feet in toward your buttocks with your feet hip-distance apart and your knees pointing to the ceiling. Rest your arms alongside your body with your palms against the floor.

2 As you breathe in, push down firmly on your hands and feet and lift your hips up as high as you can. As you breathe out, lower your hips back down to the floor. Do this five times. On the final lift, hold the posture for a few seconds and breathe deeply. Then release the pose, stretch out your legs and relax on your back.

rocking chair

This posture massages your spine and the muscles around it in a similar way to Rocking the Boat on page 34 – the difference is that, here, you rock backward and forward instead of side-to-side.

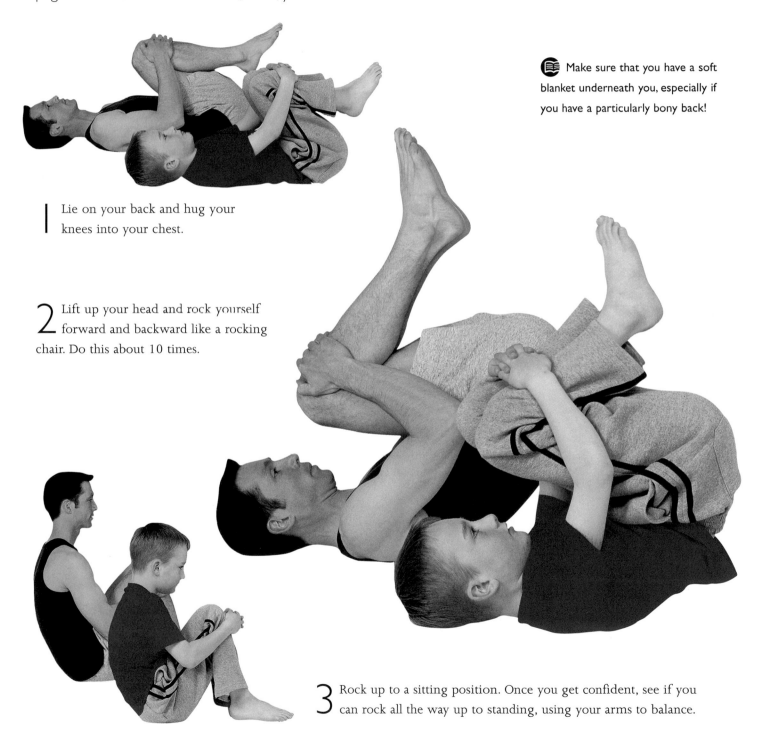

1 Lie on your back and hug your knees into your chest.

Make sure that you have a soft blanket underneath you, especially if you have a particularly bony back!

2 Lift up your head and rock yourself forward and backward like a rocking chair. Do this about 10 times.

3 Rock up to a sitting position. Once you get confident, see if you can rock all the way up to standing, using your arms to balance.

shaking it up

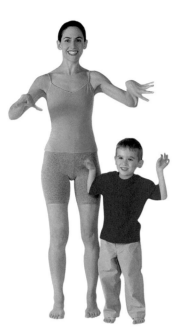

This series of movements is fantastic for getting warmed and loosened up, and for shaking out any tension or tiredness. It's also good when you're feeling stuck in a mood – you can literally shake away powerful emotions such as anger or sadness. Shaking It Up is also great fun!

1 Stand up and let yourself become loose and relaxed. Shake your hands, making your fingers and wrists as floppy as you can. Now shake your arms – your elbows first and then your shoulders.

2 Stand on your right leg and shake your left leg. Swap and shake your right leg. Now put your right foot down and shake the rest of your body – first your tummy, then your chest and then your head (gently though, to avoid getting a headache).

Try doing Shaking It Up while you sing the "Hokey Cokey" or another favourite song.

3 Now shake everything at the same time. Follow your feelings and let your body shake you – jump, dance, sing or do anything you like – let it all out! Finally, stand absolutely still and let your breathing slowly return to normal. Be aware of your entire body.

tiptoe tree and windy tree

Tiptoe Tree lengthens your spine and stretches your whole body like a terrific yawn. You can go straight into the second posture, Windy Tree, which is a dynamic sidebend that opens up the sides of your body, keeps your spine supple and tones your abdomen and digestive organs.

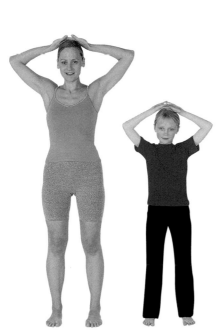

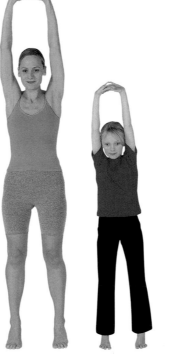

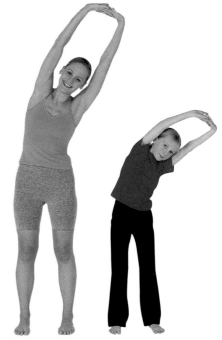

1 Stand with your feet hip-width apart and your arms by your sides. Look at a spot in front of you, keeping your gaze soft and relaxed. Interlace your fingers and put your hands on your head, palms up.

2 Breathe in deeply as you stretch your arms up high and push up onto your tiptoes (you may need to practise a few times before you can balance). This is Tiptoe Tree. Breathe out as you bring your hands back to your head and lower your heels to the floor. Do this five times, then relax.

📖 If your child finds it difficult to combine movement and breath, just focus on balancing and enjoying the stretch.

👁 Imagine that you are an enormous tree growing up toward the sky.

3 Breathe in as you stretch your arms above your head (keep your heels on the floor this time). Breathe out as you bend your body to the left. Don't lean forward or back. This is Windy Tree. Breathe in as you come back up. Breathe out as you bend to the right. Repeat five times and relax.

📖 Allow yourself to slowly move deeper into each stretch. But don't push yourself.

👁 Imagine that you are a tree being blown in the wind. Make a "ssshhh" sound, like the wind rustling through leaves.

helicopter

This is a twisting posture that tones your waist, hips and back and is exceptionally good for your spine. It also massages your abdominal organs and improves your circulation. And if you're feeling tired, Helicopter stimulates you and wakes you up.

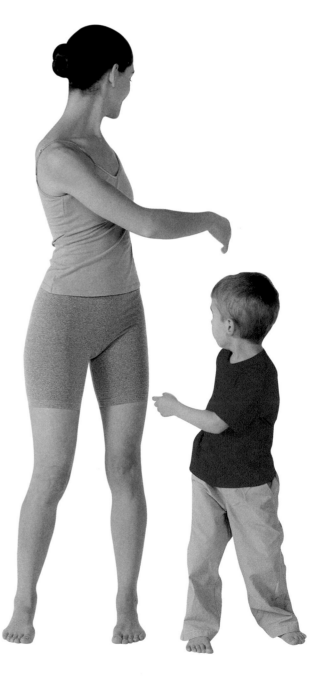

1 Stand with your feet hip-width apart or slightly wider. Stretch your arms out to the sides, palms facing down.

2 Twist to your left, taking your left hand around to the back of your right hip, your right arm around the front of your body and your right hand to your left shoulder. Look behind you. Breathe in and twist back to the centre with your arms stretched out to the sides. Now repeat the twist in the same way on the right side. Then breathe in and twist back to the centre with your arms out to the sides. Keep doing this twist and, once you've got the hang of it, start to move faster, letting your hands and arms hang loose like rags so that they swing into the position. Keep your hips still, so that the twist stays in your spine and doesn't move down into your knees. When you are moving quickly, let go of your breath and allow the movement to breathe for you.

👁 Imagine that you are a helicopter and your blades are spinning so fast that you are about to take off.

📖 This is quite a complicated movement. Make sure that you understand it and can do it yourself before you explain it to your child.

puppet

This posture is great for releasing tension and loosening up after a long day of sitting at an office or a school desk. The "ha" breath releases the stress and anxiety that we tend to carry around in the diaphragm and abdomen. It also cleanses your lungs and helps you to breathe better.

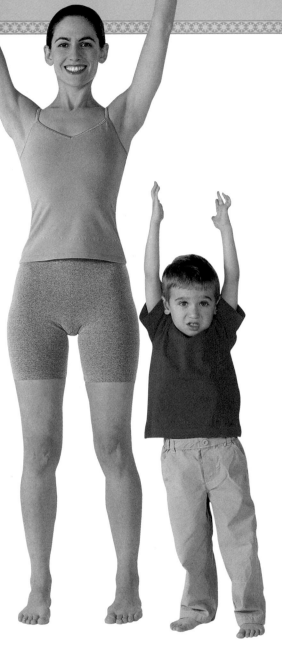

1 Stand up straight with your feet hip-width apart and your arms relaxed by your sides. As you breathe in, raise your arms above your head and stretch up as high as you can.

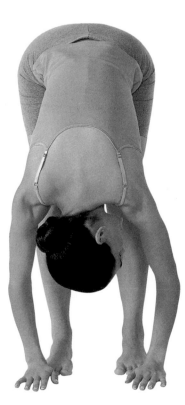

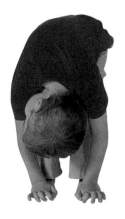

2 Breathe out as you let yourself slowly flop forward from the waist like a puppet whose strings have been cut. Keep your knees slightly bent to take the strain off your lower back and make a "haaaa!" sound as you go. Now let your arms dangle and relax your upper body and head. Rest quietly in this position, listening to your breathing. Slowly curl yourself back up to standing, keeping your arms relaxed. Bring your head up last. Do this movement several times.

the growing seed

This movement symbolizes the growth of a tiny seed into a tree. It's a wonderful way to teach children about the interaction between the earth, the sun and plant seeds. The Growing Seed helps you to get moving again if you are feeling "stuck", sluggish or heavy. It also shifts blocked energy and helps you to develop poise and muscular control.

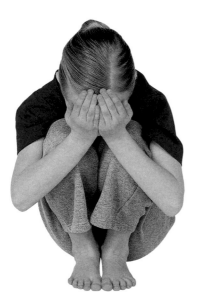

1 Squat down and curl yourself up into a little ball. Put your hands over your face so that your eyes are covered.

👁 Imagine that you are a tiny seed underneath the soil waiting for spring to come. Breathe softly and sense the earth all around you, the sound of rain pattering above you and the warmth of the sun filtering through the ground.

⇋ If you find squatting difficult, put a folded blanket underneath your heels.

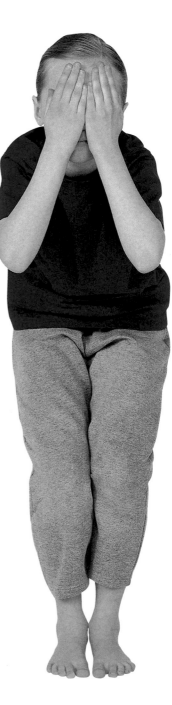

2 Start to uncurl slowly, keeping your hands over your eyes. Lift up your head and shoulders and gradually straighten your legs. Move upward like a shoot pushing toward the sun. At the moment your shoot breaks through the soil, slowly stretch your arms above your head, open your eyes wide, breathe in deeply and let out a long "ahhhhh!" sound. Repeat this cry three times, inhaling deeply after each one. Imagine all the energy of the sun streaming into you.

☺ Sprinkle a handful of mustard seeds on a damp paper towel. Put them in a warm dark place and don't let them dry out. In a few days you'll have lots of sprouts that you can eat!

📖 When we do yoga, we cultivate the seeds of peace, love and wisdom within us. Think of the practices of yoga as the tools that remove stones and plough the field, so that the seeds can grow without obstacle.

greeting the sun

Greeting the Sun is one of the most important and widely used practices in yoga. It consists of 12 postures performed in a flowing sequence in synchrony with your breath. It is good for children because it stimulates all the muscles, joints and organs and keeps the whole body working harmoniously. It also fortifies the heart and lungs and builds tremendous strength, flexibility and co-ordination.

Greeting the Sun is known as *suryanamaskar* in Sanskrit – *surya* means "sun" and *namaskar* is a respectful greeting. The best – and most traditional – time and place to practise Greeting the Sun is first thing in the morning out of doors when all the healing power of the sun's rays can be absorbed into your body. It is also wonderful to Greet the Sun at dusk when the sun is just setting in the sky. It is best to avoid practising the sequence outdoors when the sun is at its hottest or when the weather is cold.

Try to practise Greeting the Sun as mindfully (see page 21) as possible. Think about the importance of the sun and about how it provides the energy that gives us warmth and food. When you Greet the Sun in yoga imagine that you are giving thanks for the source of life on our planet. You can even paint a picture of a beautiful bright sun giving off rays of light and heat. If you practise Greeting the Sun indoors, you can put this picture in front of you to remind you what the sequence is all about.

BREAKING DOWN THE SEQUENCE

Because Greeting the Sun is quite long (see next page for the full sequence), I suggest that you teach it to your child in stages, over several yoga sessions. This way each posture receives plenty of attention and the overall sequence becomes easier to assimilate. Each of the following stages can also be practised as a mini-sequence in its own right.

STAGE ONE:
Prayer Pose – Hands Up – Standing Sandwich – Hands Up – Prayer Pose
STAGE TWO (do this part at least twice and alternate your legs in Galloping Horse):
Prayer Pose – Hands Up – Standing Sandwich – Galloping Horse – Standing Sandwich – Hands Up – Prayer Pose
STAGE THREE (alternate your legs in Galloping Horse):
Prayer Pose – Hands Up – Standing Sandwich – Galloping Horse – Face-Down Dog –
Galloping Horse – Standing Sandwich – Hands Up – Prayer Pose
STAGE FOUR:
Cat (see page 69) – Eight-Limb Salute – Cobra – Cat
STAGE FIVE:
Cat – Face-Down Dog – Eight-Limb Salute – Cobra – Face-Down Dog – Cat

the full sequence

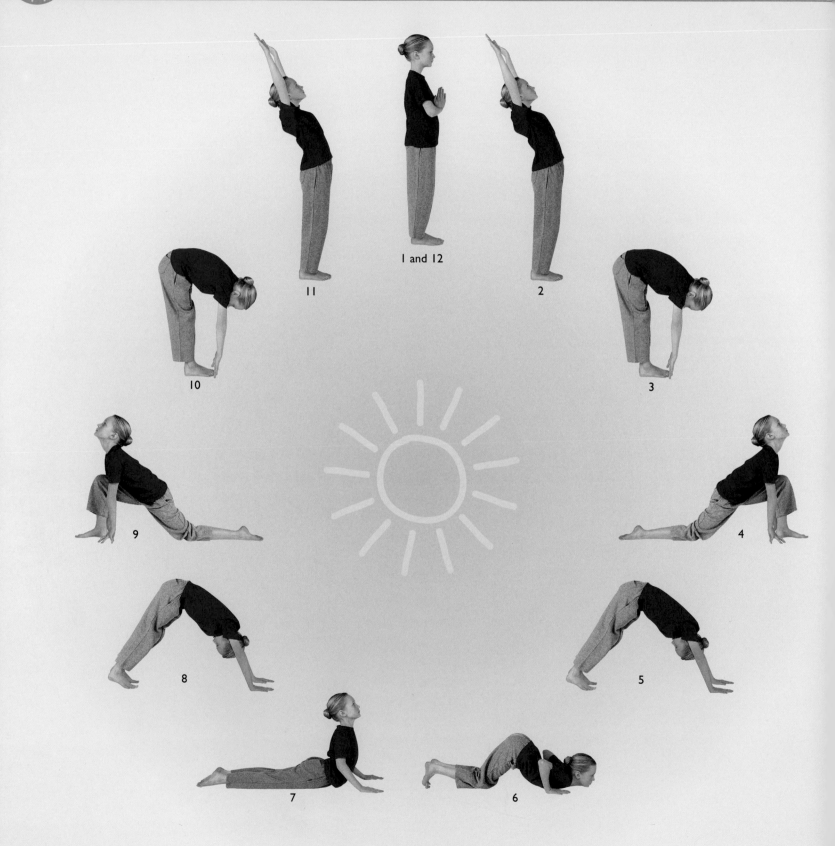

1 and 12

11

2

10

3

9

4

8

5

7

6

1. Prayer Pose

Stand up straight with your feet together. Join your palms at your heart. Keep your breathing and your body relaxed. Bring your awareness to your body.

2. Hands Up

Bring your arms forward and up above your head. Breathe in and look up toward your hands. Lean back slightly.

3. Standing Sandwich

Breathe out and bend slowly forward from your hips. Bring your head toward your knees. Put your hands or fingers on the floor or take hold of the backs of your legs.

4. The Galloping Horse

Breathe in, step back with your right leg and bring your right knee to the floor. Keep your left foot flat with your knee directly above it. Rest your fingertips on either side of your left foot and lift your chest, shoulders and head. Look up slightly.

5. Face-Down Dog

Breathe out and take your left foot back to join your right foot. Push your heels down and lift your hips high in the air. Your back and legs should be straight so that your body forms a triangle. Breathe in.

A more gentle version of Face-Down Dog is Giraffe. To do Giraffe, simply walk your feet closer to your hands after you lift your hips in the air. This is easier on your arms and shoulders.

6. Eight-Limb Salute

Breathe out and come down onto your knees, then lower your chest and chin onto the floor – your bottom should stick up in the air.

If you did Giraffe in step 5 you will need to create more space between your hands and knees in step 6.

7. Cobra

Breathe in, slide forward onto your tummy and use your back and arm muscles to lift your chest, head and shoulders up. Try to curl up like a banana while keeping the lowest part of your tummy on the floor.

From here, the postures repeat themselves in reverse order.

8. Face-Down Dog

Breathe out and push your hips back and up. Push your heels down toward the floor and keep your back and legs straight so that your body forms a triangle (as in step 5).

If you can't push straight back into Face-Down Dog, come onto your hands and knees with your hands directly under your shoulders and your knees under your hips (this is Cat; see page 69, step 1) and then move into Face-Down Dog.

9. Galloping Horse

Breathe in, step your right foot between your hands. Drop your left knee to the floor. Lift your chest, shoulders and head and look up slightly.

10. Standing Sandwich

Breathe out and step your left foot forward so that it is alongside your right foot. Straighten your legs. Keep your head as close to your knees as you can and your hands on the floor or holding the backs of your legs.

11. Hands Up

Breathe in and slowly come up to standing. Stretch your arms above your head and gently lean back.

12. Prayer Pose

Breathe out, bring your palms together in front of your heart. Rest here, noticing how your body feels before you begin the next round of Greeting the Sun. Repeat the whole sequence several times.

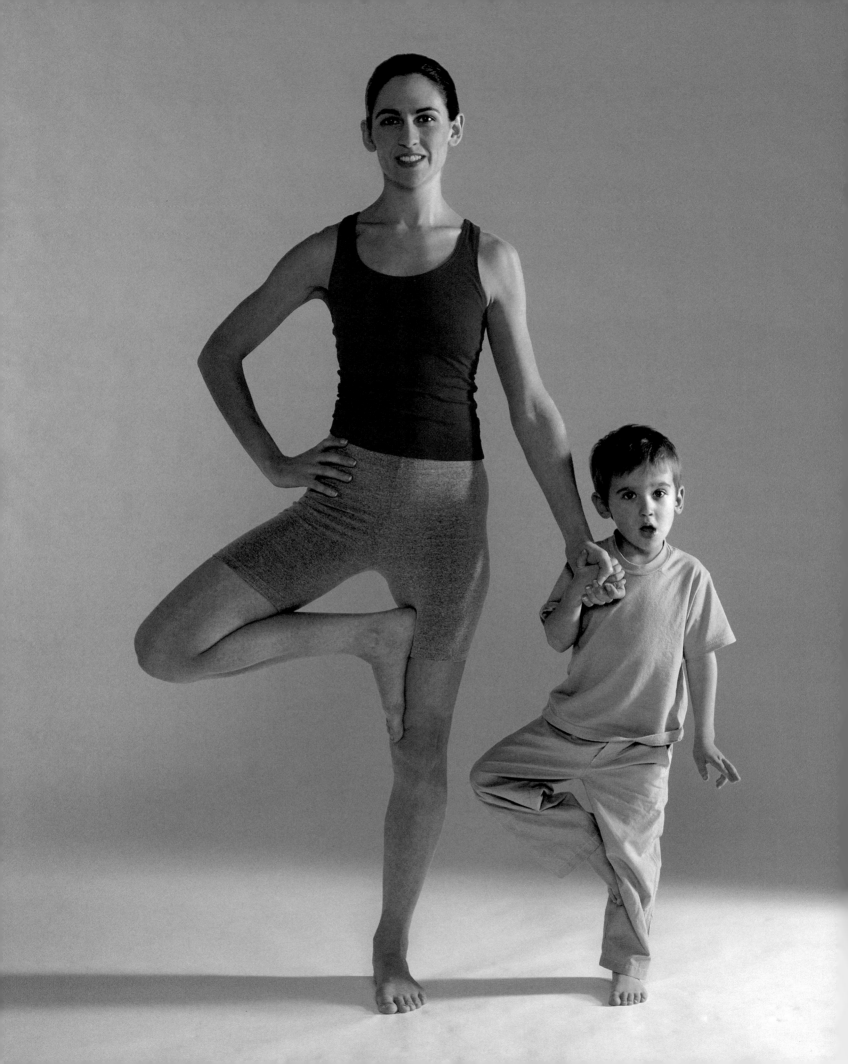

posture building blocks

This chapter consists of traditional yoga postures (*asana*) that have been practised for more than a thousand years. The ancient yogis of India knew that these postures would make their bodies healthy and strong. They also knew that the effects of each *asana* are mirrored in the mind, which itself becomes healthy, flexible and strong.

Together the postures in this chapter form a balanced and well-rounded yoga practice for you and your child. Even if you don't do every posture, or if you decide to substitute your own postures or ones from another chapter, bear in mind that any complete yoga practice should consist of at least one of each of the following: a sidebend (such as Triangle on page 50), a balancing pose (such as Tree on page 49), a forward bend (such as Sitting Sandwich on page 54), a backbend (such as Camel on page 57), a twist (such as Sailing Boat on page 56) and an inverted pose (such as Rocket on page 58).

mountain

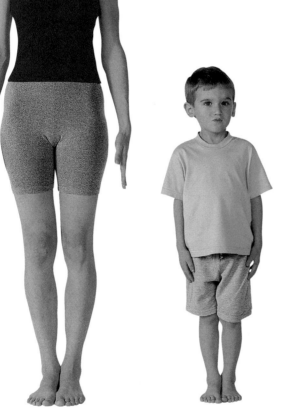

TADASANA This is the most important of all the standing poses in yoga. It teaches you how to be still and grounded and to stand as steady as a mountain. You can do Mountain at any time, whether you are lining up to go into class or waiting for a bus. It helps you to get into the habit of standing correctly and it can make you feel instantly more awake and centred.

Stand with your heels, anklebones and big toes touching. Fan your toes out across the floor. Imagine that, on each foot, there is a triangle between the ball of your big toe, the ball of your little toe and your heel. Spread your body weight evenly across these triangles. Gently pull up the muscles on the fronts of your thighs. Pull in your lower abdomen slightly and lift your chest. Roll your shoulders back and down. Keep them relaxed though – don't push them back like a soldier because this closes your lungs at the back. Your arms should be relaxed by your sides and your head should be balanced on your shoulders so that your neck muscles can relax. Become as still, steady and firm in this position as you can.

👁 Imagine that you are a mountain in the Himalayas, perhaps Mount Everest, reaching up majestically toward the sky.

☺ A mountain is silent, still and patient. Can you be these things when you stand in Mountain?

📖 **PREVENTING POSTURAL PROBLEMS**
Bad posture can come from wearing ill-fitting shoes, slouching, standing with all your weight on one leg or carrying your weight on your heels. In the long term, bad posture can result in spinal problems such as "swayback" (excessive curvature or "lordosis" of the lumbar spine), hunched back and rounded shoulders. By learning good postural habits through standing in Mountain, you will help to prevent these problems.

tree

VRICHASANA Tree is one of the classical balancing postures in yoga. It gives you poise and teaches you how to be strong and rooted without being rigid – much like a tree. You also learn to breathe slowly and deeply in harmony with the universe.

2 Find your balance, breathe in, take your arms above your head and join your palms (if you used a belt in step 1, just put your free hand on your hip). Balance here, breathing deeply and becoming still and centred. Release the pose slowly and repeat on the other side.

⇄ If joining your palms together is difficult or uncomfortable, keep your arms apart (see step 5, page 120).

⇄ When you get really good at Tree, try closing your eyes in the final stage.

👁 Imagine that you are a tall tree connecting sky and earth in the middle of a big forest. You send roots deep into the ground through your foot, and your arms and hands are branches and leaves.

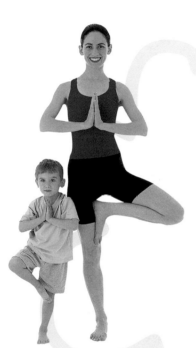

1 Stand with your feet together. Wriggle the soles of your feet into the floor to feel grounded and stable. Gaze softly at a point on the wall. Become as still in your body as possible. Lift your right foot and place the sole as high up on your left thigh as you can (if your foot keeps slipping, wear shorts or hold a belt around your ankle). If this is too difficult, place your foot on your shin instead. Join your hands at your heart.

☺ **GAMES YOU CAN PLAY USING TREE**

Get an adult to do Tree. Now fly around them like a bird, whistling and singing – see if you can get the Tree to lose its balance (no touching allowed!). Now swap.

Another game you can play is a version of Mr Wolf. You need two or more people. One person – Mr Wolf – stands facing a wall. The others stand at the other end of the room. They must creep toward Mr Wolf without waking him. If Mr Wolf hears someone coming, he shouts: "One, two, three, four, mind my teeth and mind my claws!" and jumps round. The others must do Tree – if anyone is caught with both feet on the floor they get eaten and become the new Mr Wolf.

triangle

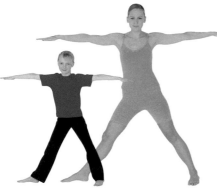

TRIKONASANA This is one of the most well known yoga postures. It stretches and tones the backs of your legs and the sides of your trunk and waist. Stability (*sthira* in Sanskrit) and ease (*sukha* in Sanskrit) are two qualities that are always important in yoga, and nowhere more so than in Triangle. A triangle is the most stable geometrical shape – to understand why, think about the stability of a camera tripod or the great pyramids of Egypt.

1 Take your feet wide apart so that there is roughly one leg-length between them – you can jump into this position if you like. Stretch your arms out to the sides, palms facing down. Turn your right foot 90 degrees to the right – facing the same direction as your right ear – and turn your left foot in slightly.

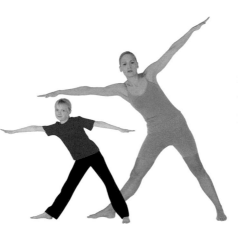

2 As you breathe out, extend to the right from your waist. Lead with your right arm. Try not to lean forward or backward.

3 Rest your right hand on your right shin or ankle. Raise your left hand in the air and, when you've got your balance, turn your chest more and look up at your left thumb. Stay here for a few moments, breathing softly and becoming steady. Breathe in as you come back up with your arms out to the sides. Now turn your left foot 90 degrees to the left and your right foot inward. Repeat the posture on the other side. You can jump or step your feet back together to finish or you can go straight on to Half Moon (see opposite).

📖 If you are very flexible, you may be able to put your hand on your foot. Don't turn your upper body toward the floor to do this. Rotate your chest up.

half moon

ARDHA CHANDRASANA Half Moon gives you a tremendous sense of balance and it tones and strengthens your legs, hips and waist. It is a challenging balance that smaller children will need plenty of assistance with. Don't worry if the first few times you try it you both end up in a heap on the floor!

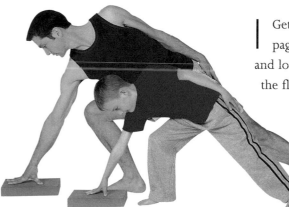

1 Get into the final stage of Triangle by following the steps on the opposite page (bend toward the right). Now bring your left arm down by your side and look at the floor. Bend your right leg and put your right hand either on the floor or on a block (or a pile of books) in front of your right foot.

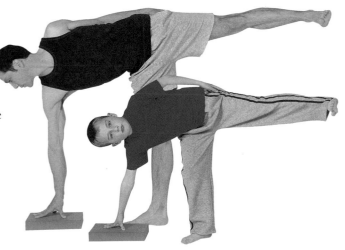

2 Hop your left leg in, take your weight on your right foot and, as you breathe in, lift your left leg in the air. Look at a fixed point on the floor or wall to steady yourself. Become as stable as you can. You can stay here before releasing the pose or you can go on to the final stage.

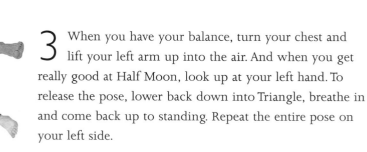

3 When you have your balance, turn your chest and lift your left arm up into the air. And when you get really good at Half Moon, look up at your left hand. To release the pose, lower back down into Triangle, breathe in and come back up to standing. Repeat the entire pose on your left side.

⊖ If your child finds this pose difficult at first, get them to do it with their back against a wall for support.

arrow

PARSVAKONASANA This pose, which is sometimes known as the "extended Triangle" (see page 50), is great for building strength and flexibility in your hips and legs. It's also very invigorating. One side of your body forms a perfectly straight line, from foot to fingertips, hence the name "arrow".

Stand with your feet together. Gently pull up the fronts of your thighs and lift your chest. Now step or jump your feet apart and stretch your arms out to the sides, palms facing down. Turn your right foot 90 degrees to the right and your left foot slightly in.

👁 Arjuna was a great Indian archer, famous for his one-pointed concentration and for never missing a target. He symbolizes the ability to aim for a goal without distraction. When you do Arrow, imagine speeding through the sky toward your target.

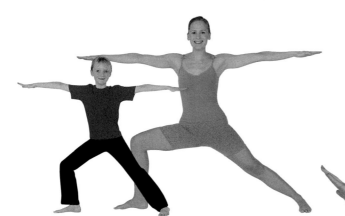

2 As you breathe out, bend your right leg so that you go into a deep lunge with your knee directly above your foot.

3 Bring your right forearm onto your right thigh. Take your left arm over your ear, so that the entire left side of your body forms a straight line. Rotate your trunk upward and look up at the ceiling along the inside of your arm. Stretch along the whole of your left side. To release the pose, breathe in, bring your left arm back and straighten your right leg. Repeat the pose on your left side, then step or jump your feet back together.

📖 Knee alignment is important in this pose to protect the joint from damage. Don't let your knee swing out to the right or the left or go beyond your foot.

warrior

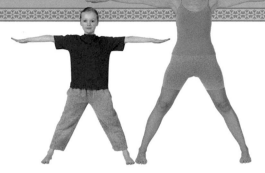

VIRABHADRASANA This posture is named after the mythical Indian warrior Virabhadra. It is especially good for strengthening your legs and back, and opening your chest.

Virabhadra was a fearsome warrior and this pose represents him lunging forward with a great sword lifted above his head. As yoga is a non-violent practice you can use this posture to give you the strength, stamina and courage to be a peaceful warrior, fighting for a better world.

1 Stand with your heels, anklebones and big toes touching. Spread your weight evenly across your feet. Gently pull up the fronts of your thighs and lift your chest. Keep your head in line with your neck. Step or jump your feet apart and stretch your arms to the sides, palms down.

2 Turn your right foot 90 degrees to the right and turn your left foot in by 45 degrees. Your left heel should be in line with the instep of your right foot. Turn your hips, chest and shoulders to face the same way as your right foot. As you breathe in, imagine lifting a big sword and raise your arms up above your head. Bring your palms together.

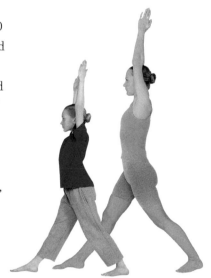

3 As you breathe out, bend your right leg so that you come into a deep lunge. Don't let your knee sway to the right or the left or go beyond your foot. Look up at your hands, lift your chest and stretch up toward the sky. Feel yourself strong and steady like Virabhadra. Breathe in deeply and, as you breathe out, make a ferocious "haaa!" sound. Warrior can be tiring, so just stay for a few seconds at first. To release the pose, straighten your right leg and lower your arms. Repeat the pose on the left side.

sitting sandwich

PASCHIMOTTANASANA This is a simple forward bend that has a profoundly soothing effect on the nervous system. In Sanskrit, *Paschimottanasana* means "intense stretch to the west". In yoga the back of the body is referred to as the west and the front of the body as the east. This is because yoga is traditionally practised as you face the rising sun in the east.

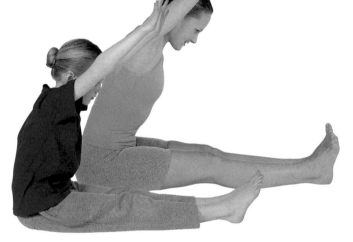

1 Sit on the floor and stretch your legs out in front of you. Make your back as straight as you can, breathe in and raise your arms above your head.

2 Breathe out, bend forward from your hips and extend your trunk forward and up. Keep your chest open and your spine long – don't collapse your chest to get your head down to your legs.

🔄 If your child is feeling tired or anxious, put pillows on their legs and get them to lean forward and rest their head – use plenty of pillows to make this comfortable. Let them stay in this position for a minute or two while you sing a soothing song or play some relaxing music. Make sure your child can breathe easily – catarrh can sometimes be a problem in this position.

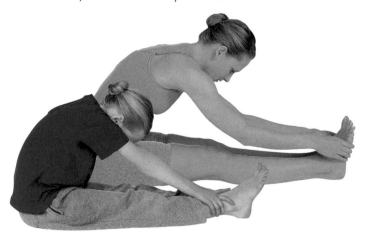

3 Breathe in, come back up to sitting, then on your next exhalation bend forward again. Do this between three and five times. On the final time grasp your feet, ankles or shins and hold this position for a few breaths. Finally, come back up to sitting and relax.

👁 Pretend that the top part of your body and your legs are slices of bread and that you have to make a sandwich by bringing them together. What filling will you put in your sandwich? Every time you sit up think of a new filling before you fold forward again.

half butterfly

This posture gives a gentle stretch to your hips and back. It also aids digestion and helps you to eliminate waste. Like Sitting Sandwich (see opposite), it is a very soothing pose.

1 Sit up straight with your legs stretched out in front of you. Bend your right leg and put the sole of your right foot against the inside of your left thigh. Your right knee should be on the floor – if it isn't, put a folded blanket under it for support. Lift your arms up above your head and stretch tall.

2 Extend forward and bring your chest and head down toward your left leg. Keep your chest lifted and open (don't collapse it to try to get lower) and your back long. Make sure that your shoulders and chest are level.

3 Take hold of your left shin or foot and relax in this position – if you like, you can rest your forehead on a pillow or a cushion and close your eyes. Sit up to release the pose and then repeat with your left leg bent.

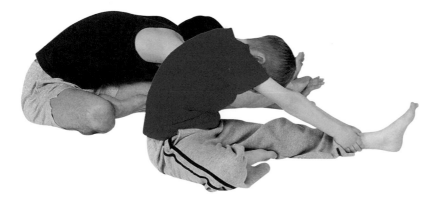

sailing boat

ARDHA MATSEYENDRASANA This classic twisting posture wrings old and stagnant blood out of your spine area – a bit like you would wring water out of a cloth – allowing fresh blood and nutrients to rush back in. It stimulates both your body and mind, and massages and stretches your inner organs.

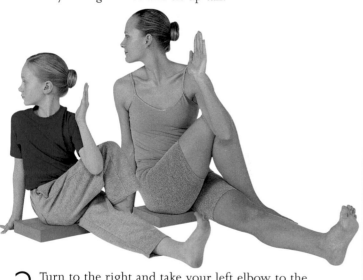

1 Sit on a cushion or a block with your legs stretched out in front of you. Bend your right leg and put your right foot on the outside of your left knee. Put your hands around your right knee and sit up tall.

2 Turn to the right and take your left elbow to the outside of your right knee with your palm facing to the right. Put your right hand on the floor behind you to balance. Twist your whole upper body to the right and look behind you. Stay in the pose for a few seconds, then release it. Straighten your legs in front of you and then repeat the twist on the other side.

👁 Pretend that you are a grand sailing boat crossing the Atlantic Ocean. How would it be in a storm when the waves are as big as houses? Or on a hot day when there is no wind to blow you along? What cargo might you be carrying in your hold? And where are you going?

📖 Because the inner organs restrict the free movement of the diaphragm during twisting postures it is more difficult to take long, smooth breaths. You should never hold your breath though – try to breathe as fully and as deeply as you can.

⇄ A more challenging variation of this twist involves feeding your left arm under your right leg, then taking your right arm around your back and clasping your fingers or wrist.

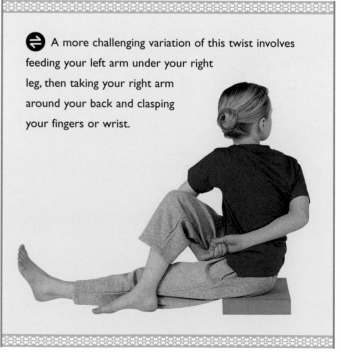

camel

USHTRASANA This backbend stretches your spine and opens out your chest and shoulders. It's good for problems such as asthma and bronchitis. The posture also corrects the tendency to hunch over, which both adults and children do when sitting at desks for long periods. Camels are symbols of endurance and self-sufficiency – in this posture, you draw upon your own reserves of patience and stamina.

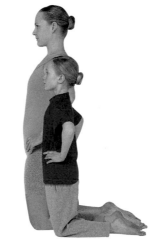

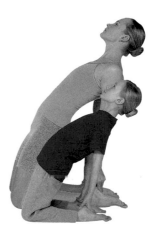

1 Kneel up with your knees and feet about hip-distance apart. Put your hands on your hips.

⮂ When you first do Camel, turn your toes under to raise your heels and make the pose easier. You can also kneel on a folded blanket.

2 Gently lean back, bringing your right hand, then your left, onto your heels. If you can't find your heels with your hands, turn and look. Then gently move your head back and gaze up.

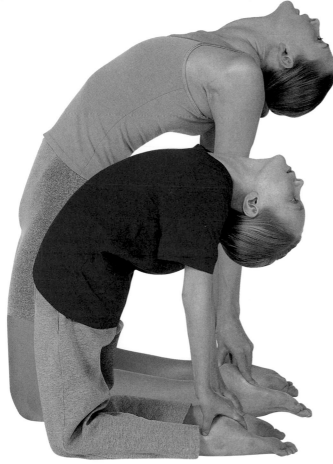

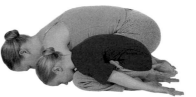

📖 Don't do Camel if you have neck problems.

4 Release your hands one at a time. Kneel down and bring your forehead forward to rest on the floor with your arms by your sides. This is called Mouse (see page 68) and it gives a gentle counter-stretch to your spine.

3 Push your hips forward so that your thighs become vertical. Lift your chest. Keep gazing up and take a couple of deep breaths.

☺ Can you imitate the slow, steady walk of a camel? The animals are sometimes called "Ships of the Desert". Imagine what it would be like to be a camel walking hundreds of miles across the desert, perhaps carrying salt or spice, or fine silk clothes.

rocket

SARVANGASANA Rocket is sometimes called the "mother of all poses" because it leaves your entire body feeling refreshed and invigorated. Inverted poses such as this counteract the effects of gravity and are an excellent way to finish your yoga session.

1 Lie on a folded blanket. Raise your legs and curl your hips off the ground, rounding your back and bringing your legs over your head. Keep your arms on the floor.

📖 Although adults can hold Rocket for as long as is comfortable, children should only hold the pose for a short time. A few seconds is enough to begin with.

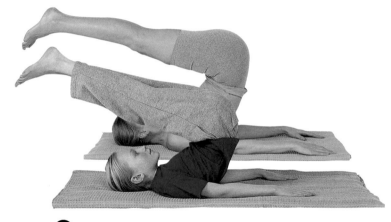

⇄ It is important to keep your neck free from pressure in this posture. Always have plenty of padding underneath your head, neck and shoulders (and elbows). If you feel any neck discomfort in Rocket, position yourself so that your shoulders are on the edge of the blanket and your head is on the floor.

2 Support your back with the palms of your hands and stretch your legs and body up toward the sky, like a rocket shooting up toward the moon. Breathe as deeply as possible and make a "shhhh" sound every time you breathe out – this naturally lengthens your exhalation and calms your mind. Stay in Rocket for as long as is comfortable, then come down the same way as you went up.

📖 Give your neck a counterstretch after Rocket. Sit up and put the middle three fingers of both hands on the back of your neck, fingertips touching. Gently move your head back for a few seconds.

👁 After Rocket, lie on your blanket with your eyes closed. Imagine that you've been rocketed out of earth's atmosphere and are floating in space. Your body is weightless. You are completely relaxed as you drift past stars, moons and planets. After a while, float down to earth on a parachute and land softly on your blanket.

TOPSY-TURVY POSE

If your child is too young to do Rocket, you can help them to get the benefits of inversion by doing this Topsy-turvy Pose together.

Alternatively, for really young children or babies, lie them along your legs with their head near your feet. Hold their hands and tip them into an inclined position by bending your legs.

You need to be quite strong (or your child needs to be quite light!) to do this pose. Be especially careful of your back. If you feel any discomfort, stop.

1 Ask your child to jump up (or pick them up) and wrap their legs around your waist. Support their hips with your hands and slowly lower them backward until they are upside down.

2 To come out of this position, get your child to put their hands on the floor and release their legs. Support their hips as they lower their legs to the floor in a slow, backward somersault.

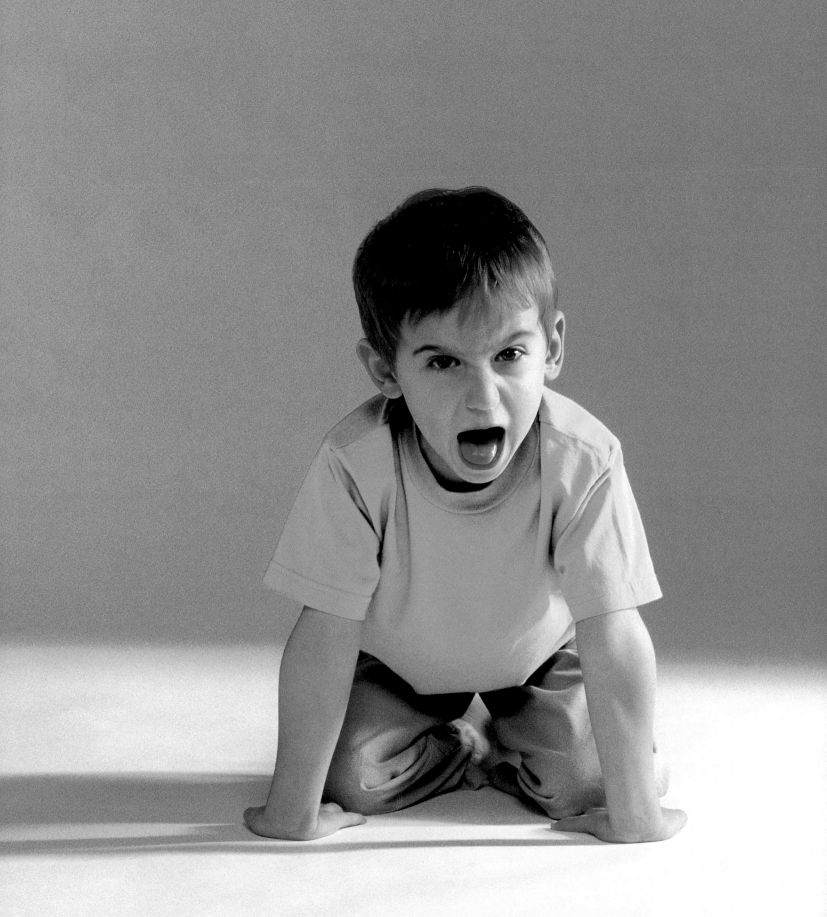

animal magic

Children love animals, and this chapter explores some of the many yoga postures that are based on birds and beasts. The ancient yogis of India lived deep in the forest, far away from people or towns, and had plenty of time to study nature. They found that by impersonating certain animals, they could acquire the strengths and gifts possessed by them. For example, by imitating a lion, their voices became clear and strong, and by copying a snake, their spines became free and flexible.

Each posture in this chapter has its own unique benefits for your body and mind. It's also great fun just to get inside the skin of an animal and imagine how it feels to be, say, a mouse, lion or pigeon. Encourage your child to let their imagination run wild. Make up your own postures based on animals that your child has seen or read about. Imitate the noises of the animals and imagine what they would say if they could talk. You can even dress up as your favourite animal.

albatross

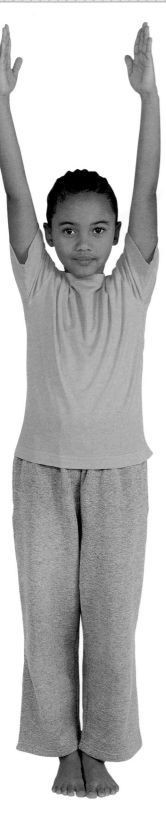

This simple posture can have profound effects if you do it slowly and with mindfulness. By synchronizing your breath with the movement of your arms, you bring your body and mind into harmony and become focused and centred. Albatross is also a good practical way to prepare yourself for the breathing exercises in Chapter 6.

1 Stand with your anklebones and big toes touching. Spread your body weight evenly across the soles of your feet and gently pull up the muscles on the fronts of your thighs. Roll your shoulders back and down, but keep them relaxed. Keep your arms straight down by your sides and your head and neck relaxed. Become as still, steady and firm in this position as you can. Now, as you breathe in, slowly lift your arms to the sides and above your head.

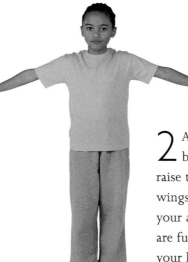

2 As you breathe out, slowly bring your arms back down to your sides. As you breathe in, raise them again – as if your arms are huge wings. Keep doing this, making sure that when your arms are at their highest point, your lungs are full, and when your arms are by your sides, your lungs are empty. Make your movements as slow and graceful as you can.

👁 Imagine that you are a magnificent albatross standing on a rock overlooking the ocean. You are getting ready for a long voyage. As you take off, picture yourself flapping your enormous wings as you fly majestically over the waves.

📖 If your child needs to breathe faster, get them to flap their wings a bit faster, too. For very small children, synchronizing breathing and movement might be too difficult, in which case just let them enjoy flapping like a big bird.

cockerel

This is another simple exercise that links breath with movement and helps you to breathe deeply and fully. The emphasis here is on lengthening your exhalations – something which calms your mind. Each time you exhale, you make the sound of a cockerel waking up in the morning.

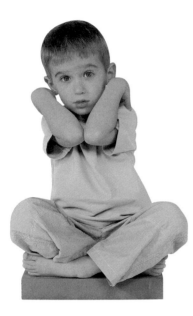

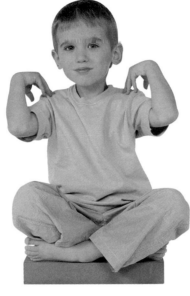

Imagine that you have a pair of brilliant red, black and gold wings that are shining in the morning sun.

1 Sit on a cushion or block, put your fingertips on your shoulders and bring your elbows together in front of your body. These are your cockerel wings.

2 Take your elbows apart and then up, using them to draw big circles in the air. Breathe in on the upward part of the movement and out on the downward part of the movement. Now change the direction of your circles.

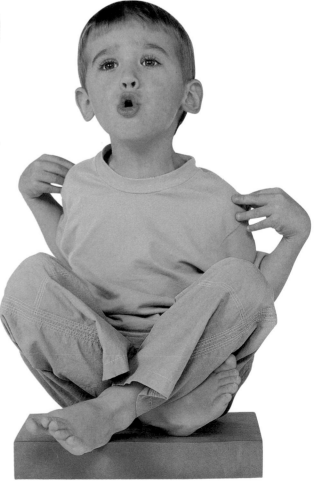

3 When you've practised combining breath and movement a few times, try crowing like a cockerel, "cock-a-doodle-dooo", on your out-breath. Make the "oooo" sound as long as possible. Repeat this exercise several times, but don't strain – keep your breath and movements comfortable.

pigeon king

This backbending posture makes your hips flexible and strengthens the muscles in your back and neck. Your chest is fully expanded, allowing you to breathe deeply and fully. Pigeon King is also good for the health of your urinary tract.

1 Kneel on all fours, hands directly under your shoulders and knees under your hips. Support yourself with your hands, slide your right knee forward and your right foot across your left knee so that you rest on the outside of your right shin. Slide your left leg back until it is flat on the floor. Ideally your right ankle should touch your left hip bone. Put a cushion or block under your right buttock if your hips are in the air.

2 Lift up your chest and gently arch your back. Look up and breathe. This is the first stage of Pigeon King. Hold it for a few seconds.

☺ Everyone knows what pigeons look like, but did you know that pigeons were once used to deliver messages hundreds of miles away, much like we use email today? Pigeons have a fantastic sense of direction and are very strong fliers. When you do Pigeon King, really puff out your chest like a proud pigeon who has just delivered an important message.

3 Walk your hands forward and lay your forehead on the floor. This is the second stage of Pigeon King – it can be very soothing, especially if you coo softly to yourself like a pigeon. Finally, walk your hands back in and come back onto all fours. Repeat the posture on the left side.

eagle

This is a balancing posture that develops your concentration and focus. It strengthens the joints and muscles in your legs and gets rid of any stiffness in your shoulders and upper back.

1 Stand up straight with your feet together. Become as still, steady and firm as you can. Find a point on the wall in front of you and gaze at it softly. Raise your left arm in front of you, palm up. Bring your right arm underneath, so that your arms cross at the elbows.

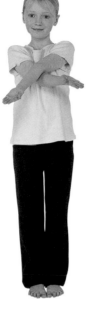

2 Bend your left arm so that your forearm is vertical, with the palm facing to the right. Then bend your right arm and entwine it around your left arm. Try to join your palms together.

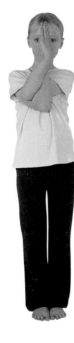

3 Keeping your arms entwined, bend your knees and wrap your right leg around the front of your left leg. Your right foot should hook around the inside of your left ankle. (This is quite a complicated manoeuvre – in the beginning just standing on one leg is fine.) Now unwind your arms and your legs and repeat the pose on the other side.

When you are learning Eagle, do step 2 on its own, then relax your arms and try entwining your legs in step 3. Later on you can put both stages together.

Imagine that you are an eagle perched on a craggy rock, keeping watch over the land.

Eagles are known for their incredible vision and strength – they symbolize the ability to see our goals clearly and the power to accomplish them. Look at pictures of eagles in library books or go to a bird sanctuary that keeps birds of prey. You can also try imitating the cry of the eagle and soaring around the room looking for prey. Every so often, come back to your perch and get into Eagle. As you "unspiral" out of the pose, soar away once more.

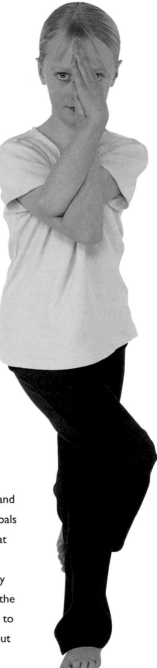

lion

This pose in which you imitate a lion's roar is great fun and is particularly good for you because it helps to keep your tonsils and throat healthy. It builds a strong voice and gives confidence in speaking and singing. In fact, sometimes Lion is used as a remedy for stammering. It's also a great way to relieve tension!

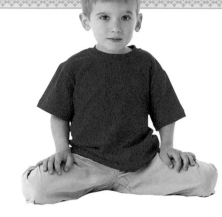

1 Kneel on the floor, separate your knees and sit back on your heels. Your big toes should be touching.

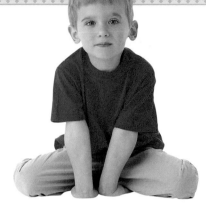

2 Gently lean forward, keeping your buttocks on your heels. Put your hands on the floor with your fingers pointing in toward your body.

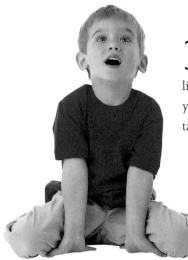

3 Make your back as long as you can and lift up your chest. Tilt your head right back and take a deep breath in.

4 Open your mouth as wide as you possibly can and stick out your tongue. See if you can get your tongue to touch your chin. Then, as you breathe out, let out a long, steady, fierce roar: "aaaaarrrrgghh!". Be careful not to strain your voice though.

☺ Get into Lion and ask your mum or dad to feed you. Surprise them by saying "thanks" with a big roar.

kicking mule

This is a dynamic posture, which is a preparation for a full handstand or "Face-Down Tree", as it is called in yoga. Kicking Mule strengthens your arms and shoulders and sends plenty of fresh blood to your brain, which improves memory, learning and general vitality.

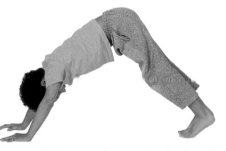

1 Come onto all fours with your hands shoulder-width apart. Tuck your toes underneath you and push your hips back and up as high as possible so that your back and legs form a triangle shape. Push your heels down toward the floor.

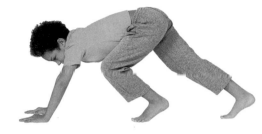

2 Step your left foot forward by about 30 cm (12 in) and shift your weight toward your hands.

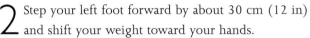

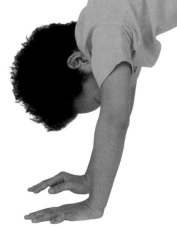

3 Push away with your left foot and kick up into the air with your right leg. Do this a few times, then swap feet and kick your left leg up into the air.

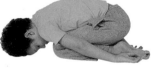

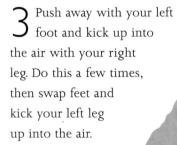

4 Relax for a minute or two by kneeling with your forehead on the floor and your arms by your sides in Mouse (see page 68).

When you've had lots of practice doing Kicking Mule, try doing a full handstand (Face-Down Tree). Start by kicking up against a wall. It can help to get a partner to support you in the pose or to hold your ankles to take some of the weight off your hands, arms and shoulders.

mouse

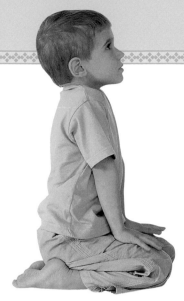

This beautiful posture, sometimes called "Child's Pose", is great for settling you down when you feel hyper or over-tired. It's also a good way to relax at the end of a yoga session or after upside-down poses such as Kicking Mule (see page 67) or Rocket (see page 58). Mouse restores energy, calms your mind and can help you to sleep.

1 Sit on your heels with your knees together and your hands on your thighs. This posture can also be used for meditation – it is called "Diamond Pose" (*Vajrasana*).

2 Put your hands on the floor in front of you. Use them for support as you lean forward and rest your forehead on the floor. If this is uncomfortable, put a pillow or a block under your forehead. Relax your arms by your sides, palms up. Stay here for a minute or two, observing your breath. Release the pose slowly, lifting your head up last. Sit on your heels while you get used to being upright again.

👁 There's a mouse in the house! Imagine that it's winter and you're curled up and ready for sleep in your cosy hole. Be as still and quiet as you can.

🙂 MAKING THE FIRE

Try doing this exercise in which you pretend that you're blowing on a small fire to help the flames grow. (Did you know that before we had electric and gas cookers, people used to make their food on real fires, and that people still cook like this in many parts of the world?)

Get into Mouse but, instead of resting your arms by your sides, put your hands and elbows on the floor in front of you. Now lift up your head and imagine that, a little way in front of you, is a small fire. You must get it going by blowing gently on it. So breathe in, pucker your lips as if you were going to whistle, and slowly and gently breathe out onto the fire. Do this five times and then rest in Mouse.

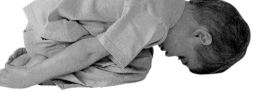

cat

This simple dynamic pose loosens up your neck, shoulders and spine. It also teaches you how to synchronize your movements with your breath.

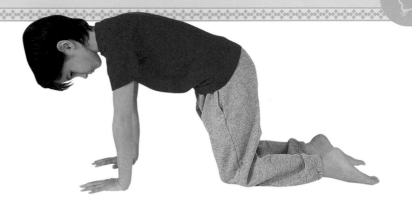

I Come onto your hands and knees, with your hands directly under your shoulders and your knees under your hips. Make your back as flat as you can. This is the starting position.

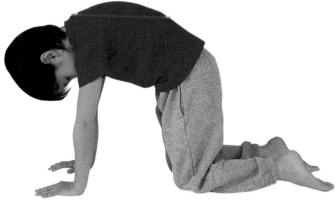

2 As you breathe out, lift your back up as high as you can and push down into your arms, rounding your back and dropping your head down. This is "angry Cat", the first position.

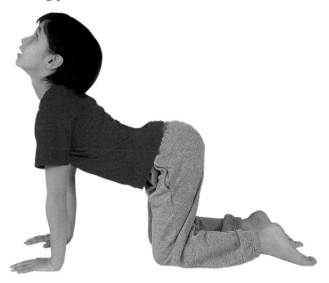

3 Breathe in, tilt your pelvis forward and push your belly button toward the floor. Hollow your back, move your head right back and look up. This is "happy Cat", the second position. Repeat steps 2 and 3 several times, taking care to match the movement of your body with your breath. When you breathe out, try miaowing like a cat, making the sound last as long as possible.

☺ Have you ever watched a cat stretch after it wakes up from a long sleep? It pushes its back in the air and then it hollows its back to stretch its spine the opposite way. These are the two movements that you copy when you do angry Cat and happy Cat.

📖 MOUSE, CAT AND DOG

You can do Mouse (see opposite), Cat and Face-Down Dog (see pages 44–5) as a mini-sequence. Start in Mouse then come onto all fours for Cat. Push up into Face-Down Dog by lifting your hips in the air so that your body forms a triangle. Now do the sequence in reverse. Repeat as many times as you like. You can even add sounds: squeak in Mouse, miaow in Cat and bark in Face-Down Dog.

snake

This posture, in which you imitate a snake lifting up its head, makes your back strong and supple. It is particularly good for you if you suffer from asthma or other respiratory disorders, because it strengthens your diaphragm (the primary muscle used in respiration – and often underused by asthma sufferers) and helps to expel carbon dioxide from your body.

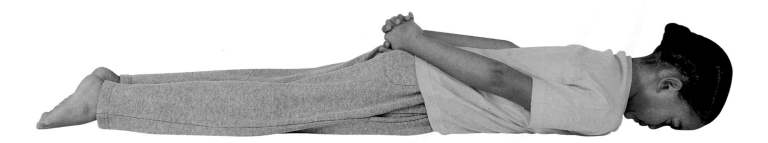

Lie on your front and rest your forehead on the floor. Bring your palms together and interlace your fingers behind your back. Become as still and centred as you can.

2 As you breathe in, stretch your arms back and lift your head, neck and chest off the floor – go as high as you can without straining. As you breathe out, lower your chest, neck and head back down to the floor. Repeat this movement a few more times. Hiss like a snake on each downward movement. Now release your arms and rest your head on your hands. Then sit on your heels and bring your forehead forward to rest on the floor with your arms by your sides. This is called Mouse (see page 68) and it gives your spine a gentle counterstretch.

👁 Think about the qualities of a snake when you do this posture. Snakes are shy and retiring creatures. They also have incredibly flexible spines.

mosquito

This posture imitates the movement of a mosquito as it moves toward its prey. The forward bend keeps your legs, hips and back flexible, and gently tones your abdomen. The position of your arms and hands prevents your shoulders from becoming rounded and helps you to breathe fully.

1 Stand with your heels, anklebones and big toes touching, bring your hands behind your back and move your shoulders down and your elbows back. Join your palms together with your fingers pointing up. Wriggle your hands up between your shoulder blades.

⇌ If you find it difficult to make your palms meet behind your back, take hold of your elbows behind your back instead. This is more gentle on your wrists and shoulders.

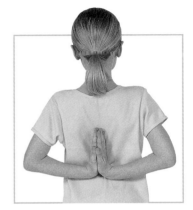

2 Turn your left foot 45 degrees away from your right foot. Take a big step forward with your right foot, keeping your shoulders, chest and hips facing forward. Find your balance, breathe in and, as you breathe out, bend forward from your hips. Now breathe in and come back up. Repeat this movement two or three times, then do the pose on the other side.

😊 Mosquitoes live by sucking the blood of humans and animals. Perhaps you've been bitten by one. As you bend forward, make a buzzing sound like a mosquito about to bite. As you come back up to standing make a sucking, "schlurping" sound like a mosquito sucking blood.

📖 Mosquito can be quite a difficult posture for small children. If your child is having trouble balancing, get them to release their arms and rest their hands on the floor, or on blocks or piles of books placed either side of their front foot.

little butterfly

This posture is a favourite among kids. It keeps the hips open and flexible and the whole pelvis and abdomen healthy. The forward bend part of the posture also gives the back a lovely, invigorating stretch.

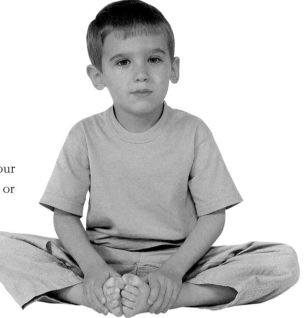

1 Sit on the floor and draw the soles of your feet together. Bring your heels as close into your body as you can and hold onto your feet or ankles. Sit up straight and tall.

⇄ If you find it difficult to keep your back straight, sit on the edge of a folded blanket or a block.

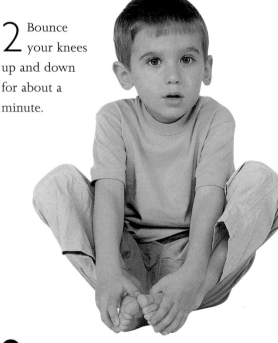

2 Bounce your knees up and down for about a minute.

👁 Imagine that your legs are the wings of a brightly coloured butterfly playing in a meadow full of flowers on a summer's day. When you do the forward bend part of the posture pretend that you are a butterfly leaning over to eat the pollen from a flower.

☺ What colours would you be if you were a butterfly? Would you have stripes, spots or star patterns on your wings? Draw a picture of yourself. What sort of flowers would you land on? What colour? Do they smell nice? Draw them too.

3 Extend gently forward from your hips, keeping your back as straight as you can. When you can't go any further, let your back gently curve over. Don't pull on your feet as this stresses your ankle joints. Stay here for a few seconds, then come back up and stretch out your legs.

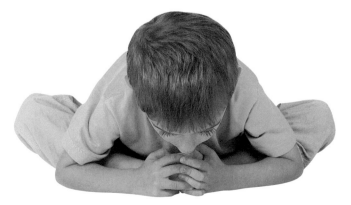

big butterfly

This is a balancing posture that you can go straight into from Little Butterfly. It usually takes some practice before you get the hang of it – keep trying though because it's a great feeling when you get your balance.

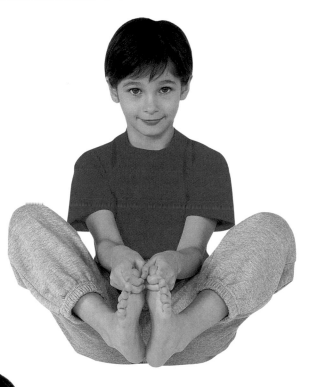

1 Do step 1 of Little Butterfly (see opposite) and then take hold of your big toes with your index and middle fingers. Balance on the part of your pelvis between your sitting bones and your tailbone. Now gently lift up your feet.

2 Slowly straighten out your legs – don't worry if they're a little bent though. Try to balance in this position with a straight back. Make sure that there is something soft behind you as you'll probably roll back a few times at first.

spider

This squatting posture is great for your feet, ankles and hips. In societies where people squat to cook, chat and go to the toilet, hip problems in later life are virtually non-existent. In Spider, the position of your hands makes your abdomen contract slightly and this not only strengthens the muscles in this area but aids digestion and elimination. The final stage of Spider is quite a challenging balance that strengthens your hands, wrists and arms and increases the effect of the pose on your abdominal muscles.

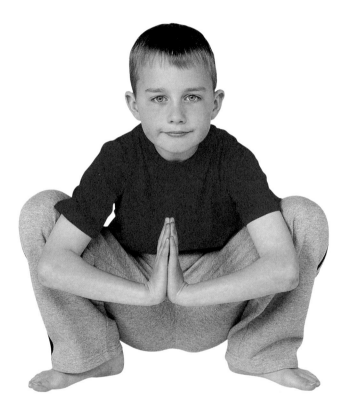

1 Stand with your feet about shoulder-width apart. Bend your knees and come into a squatting position. Join your palms together and use your elbows to push your knees wider apart. Stay in this position for a few breaths.

⇄ If it is difficult to squat with your feet flat, put a folded blanket or a block underneath your heels. A block or a folded blanket at the base of your wrists is also useful – because of the way that children's bodies develop, your arms may not be long enough to enable you to press your hands firmly on the floor.

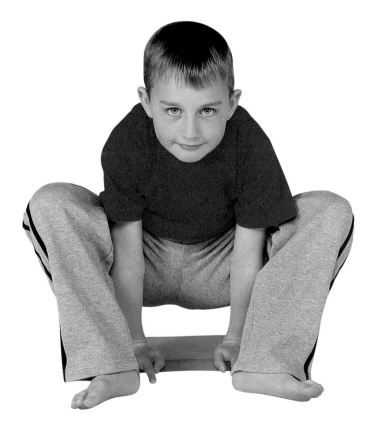

2 Release your hands, lean forward and, raising your hips a little, stretch your arms back through your legs. Put your hands on the floor behind your feet with your fingers pointing forward and your elbows slightly bent. Lower your body until you are "sitting" on your upper arms. This is the first stage of Spider – stop here if you want to.

3 Shift your weight back onto your hands, and shuffle your feet forward until you feel them lifting off the floor. Try to balance on your hands in this position.

👁 Imagine that you are a spider balancing in the middle of a huge web.

📖 Spider takes practice – be prepared to roll backward!

☺ Watch out, watch out, there's a spider about! Do the spider walk by shuffling your hands and feet around in Step 2. Get someone else to be a different kind of insect such as Dead Bug (see page 34) or Mosquito (see page 71). Can you catch them in your web?

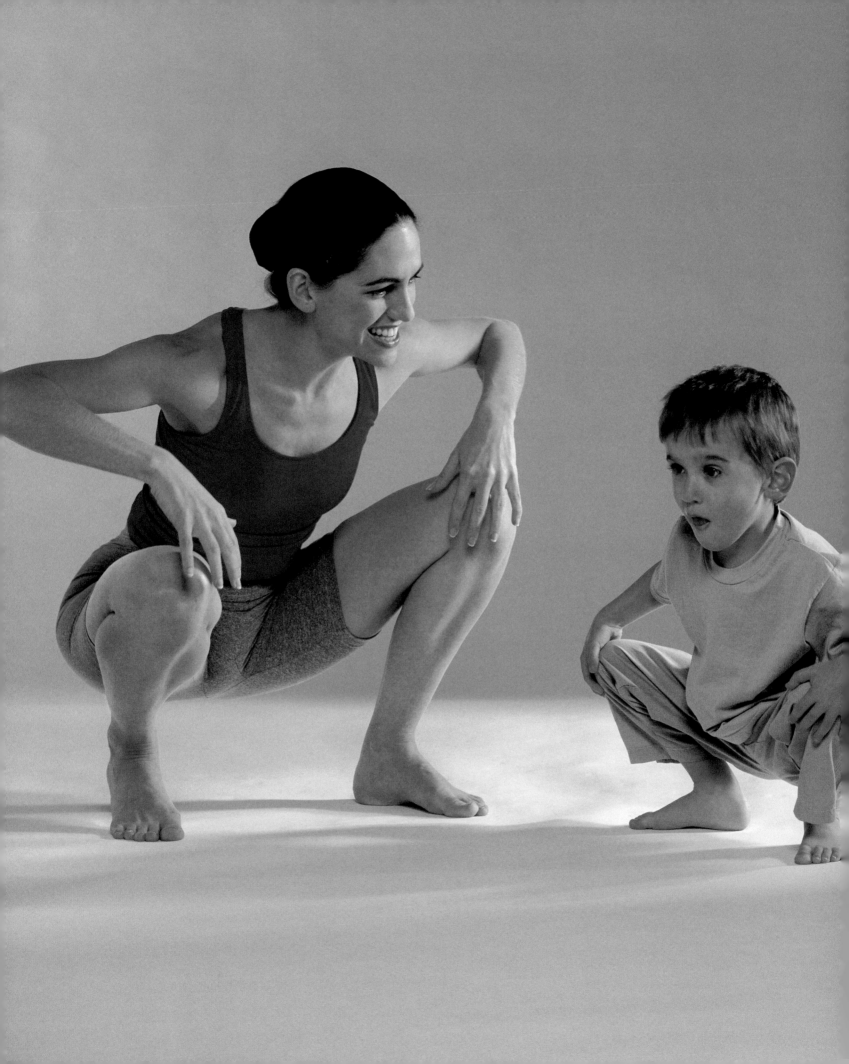

activities, journeys and games

Yoga with kids is all about imagination and creativity, and this chapter is full of ideas about how to make yoga into an exciting voyage of discovery. The postures at the beginning of the chapter are activities, such as stirring pudding or chopping wood, that you can weave into a story or an adventure. Then there are lots of quirky ways of moving around using everything from Bunny Hops to Crab Walking. In combination with the animal postures in Chapter 4, you have all the elements you need to go on safari, climb a mountain or swim up a river! The chapter ends with a selection of yoga-based team games.

How many and what type of games and activities your child is interested in will depend on their age. Young children love imaginative fantasy games whereas older children tend to be more interested in the yoga postures themselves. Try to adapt your yoga sessions to your child's individual needs and preferences.

sorting the rice

In this pose, you pretend that you're sorting a pile of rice into good grains and bad grains as you stretch forward first to one foot and then the other. The benefits of Sorting the Rice include keeping your whole pelvic area healthy and supplied with fresh blood, increasing the flexibility of the backs of your legs and stretching and toning your lower back and waist.

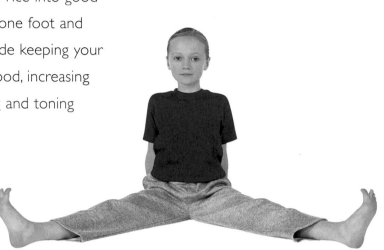

If you like, you can use sweets in this exercise. Mix a pile of two different colours and sort them by colour. You can also use two different types of dried bean.

Sit on the floor and spread your legs as far as they'll comfortably go. Sit up straight, put your hands behind you for support and lift your spine. If this is difficult, sit on a block or a cushion. Take a couple of breaths.

Be careful not to strain the insides of your knees in this pose. If you can't reach as far as your foot, just put the grains by your knee or shin.

Did you know that rice grows in extremely wet fields called paddies? In Asia rice is one of the most important foods and many people eat it every day of their lives.

2 Keeping your back straight, reach forward and pick up a grain of rice from an imaginary pile between your feet. If it's a good grain, stretch over and put it by your right foot. If it's a bad grain, stretch over and put it by your left foot. Now pluck another grain from the pile and repeat the action until there are no grains left.

stirring the pudding

Now that you've sorted the rice, it's time to make rice pudding. In this pose you make big circular stirring movements using the whole of your upper body. The benefits are the same as for Sorting the Rice. You can do the two poses in sequence.

1 Sit in the same position as for Sorting the Rice (see opposite) with your legs wide and your back straight. Take a real or imaginary wooden spoon in both hands.

👁 Picture a big cauldron full of rice pudding in front of you. It needs lots of stirring so that it doesn't get lumpy.

2 Stir the pudding by reaching out toward your left foot and making a big semi-circle with the whole of your upper body over to your right foot. The pudding is very thick, so you have to move slowly. Keep the circular motion going by leaning back and stirring the edge of the cauldron that's nearest to you, then reach out again toward your left foot. Do three of these clockwise circles then go anti-clockwise three times.

👁 Imagine that you are making a delicious Indian dish called *khir* which is made from rice, nuts, dried fruit and milk. *Khir* was the food that was given to the Buddha by a young girl when he was close to starving to death. Thanks to this act of kindness, he gained the strength to go on and attain enlightenment just a few miles from where he was sitting.

chopping the wood

This squatting pose keeps your hips and lower back healthy. In parts of Asia and Africa, where people squat instead of sitting on chairs, back problems are rare. Squatting also massages your abdominal organs and helps you to eliminate food – this is why many people find squatting an ideal position for going to the toilet. The "chopping" action works the deep muscles between your shoulder blades and prevents your shoulders from becoming hunched and rounded. The "ha" sound cleanses your lungs and throat.

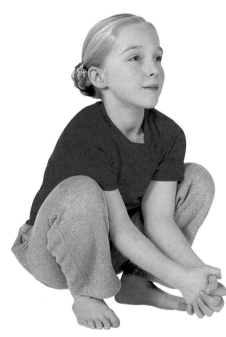

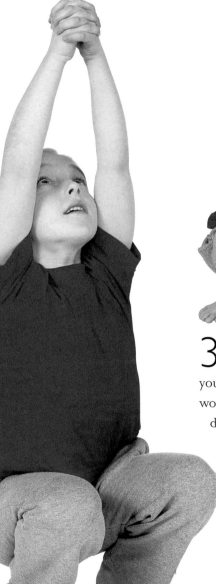

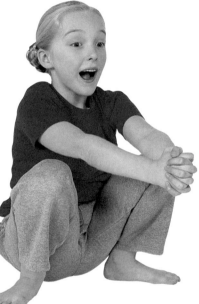

1 Stand with your feet hip-width apart and squat down, keeping your heels on the floor. If you find this difficult, try moving your feet a little further apart. If your heels don't touch the ground, put a folded blanket under them.

2 Take hold of your imaginary axe by bringing your palms together and interlacing your fingers. Raise your arms high over your head and make your spine as long as you can. Look up toward your hands.

3 As you breathe out, bring your arms quickly down in front of you as if you are chopping a piece of wood – make the sound "ha" as you do so. Raise your axe again and repeat this chopping movement about five times.

cradling the baby

This is a fantastic posture for keeping your hips and knees flexible. It also helps stagnant blood in your legs return to your heart, where it can be replenished with oxygen.

I Sit on the floor with your legs stretched out in front of you and your feet together. Put your hands behind you for support and make your back straight and tall.

2 Bend your right leg. Lift your right foot up, and using your left arm draw it across your body. Rest it in the crook of your left elbow. Wrap your right arm around your right knee and catch your left hand with your right. Stay in this position for a few breaths. Keep your back straight – if this is difficult, sit on a cushion or two. Now gently rock your right leg from left to right. Do this for as long as is comfortable then release the pose and repeat on your left leg.

If you can't cradle your foot and knee in your elbows, use your hands to support your knee and your foot instead.

Imagine that you are rocking a beautiful little baby in your arms. You can even sing a lullaby if you like.

rowing the boat

This exercise has many benefits. The forward rowing motion opens your hamstrings and the back of your body, as well as massaging your abdominal organs and muscles. The backward rowing movement strengthens your back and abdominal muscles which, together, resist the pull of gravity. Your arm movements keep your shoulder and upper back muscles free.

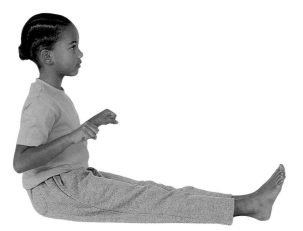

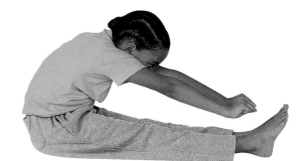

1 Sit on the floor with your legs stretched out in front of you and your ankles touching. Make fists with your hands as if you are holding the oars of a boat.

2 Lift your arms up above your head, then lean forward from your hips toward your feet, keeping your back as straight as you can.

3 When you have gone as far as you can with the forward movement, slowly pull your arms in toward you and lean back like a rower heaving their oars. When you have leaned back as far as you can, raise your arms over your head and repeat the forward rowing movement. Do the whole movement three to five times. Once you've got the hang of the exercise, breathe out on the forward movement and breathe in on the backward movement.

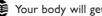

Your body will get the maximum benefit if you do this exercise very slowly.

Pretend that you are rowing across a wide lake or even an ocean. What kind of birds and animals can you see from your boat? Are there any fish in the water? Can you feel any wind? Are there waves rocking your boat?

cycling

This pose keeps your hips and knees healthy and strengthens your stomach and lower back muscles. It is also a gentle inversion which refreshes your brain with fresh, oxygen-rich blood, as well as draining stagnant blood from your legs.

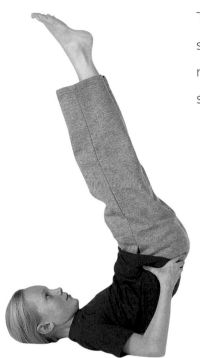

To help you to get the hang of this exercise start by moving one leg at a time.

1 Lie down on your back and gently swing your legs up so that your hips come off the floor – support your hips with your hands. If this is difficult, do the exercise with your back flat on the floor and only your legs raised.

2 Slowly start to move your legs in big circular movements, as if you are pedalling a bike. Do five complete pedals forward and five backward, then come down to a lying position and relax.

Go on an imaginary bicycling adventure. Choose a place that you'd like to visit – maybe the Sahara desert, a rainforest full of exotic animals, or Disneyland. Think about all the interesting characters that you might meet along the way. Remember, when you have a hill to climb, pedal very slowly, then, when you get over the top of the hill, cycle as fast as you can all the way down to the bottom.

building a bridge

This posture makes your spine extremely supple, and like all backbends, it brings you energy. It's a great posture to include in your yoga practice if you are feeling tired or listless and need reviving.

1 Lie on your back, bend your knees and put your feet hip-width apart on the floor. Your knees should point toward the ceiling and your arms should rest by your sides.

📖 Warm up by doing the postures in Chapter 2 before you try this pose. Building a Bridge takes a lot of strength and concentration, so don't worry if it you can't do it immediately. An easier version of the pose is Dynamic Easy Bridge on page 36.

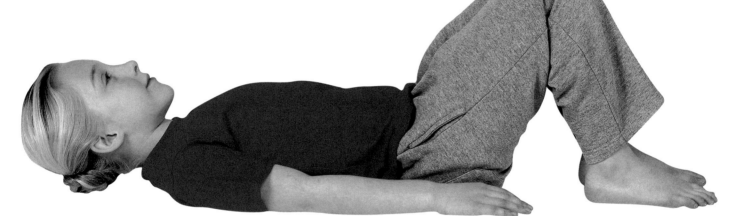

2 Put your hands under your shoulders so that your fingers point down toward your feet. Keep your arms and legs parallel – don't let your elbows or your knees splay out to the sides.

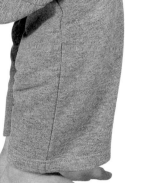

3 As you breathe out, raise your body and rest the crown of your head on the floor. This is the first stage of Building a Bridge. If you feel any pain or discomfort in your neck, stop.

4 Take another breath or two, then push up with your arms and legs so that your body forms a graceful arch and you are resting only on your hands and feet. (If you do this pose with a partner, you can take turns pretending to be fishes swimming under the bridge.) Come down by lowering yourself onto the crown of your head and then gently lying back down on the floor and resting.

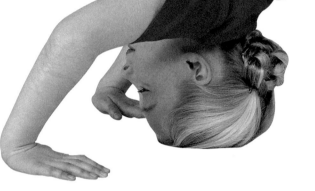 Imagine that you are a huge stone bridge spanning a mighty river.

walking the dog

This is based on Face-Down Dog (see pages 44–5) which develops great strength in your arms, shoulders and back, and improves your co-ordination. Because your head is lower than your hips, fresh blood is sent to your brain, which has a nourishing effect on your body and mind.

I Come onto all fours with your hands shoulder-width apart. Tuck your toes underneath you and push your hips back and up as high as possible so that your body forms a triangle. Push your heels down toward the floor. This is Face-Down Dog. Now walk around in this pose.

⇌ If you find Walking the Dog difficult, try Walking the Giraffe instead. Get into Face-Down Dog but move your hands and feet closer together – this takes the strain off your arms and shoulders (although it may be more challenging on your hamstrings).

👁 As you raise your leg in the air, pretend that you are a dog spraying a post to mark your territory. Imagine that you're walking down a street spraying each post that you come to. Make barking and panting noises as you go.

2 When you've got used to walking in Face-Down Dog, try doing this on-the-spot exercise: lift up first your right leg and then your left leg as high as you can.

toad walking

As with all squats, Toad Walking loosens up your hips and lower back, and tones your whole pelvic area. It also builds strength in your leg muscles and massages your inner organs. The insect-catching part of the exercise develops and relaxes your tongue and eye muscles.

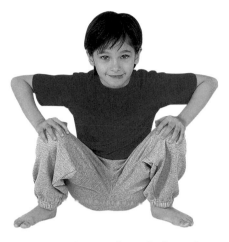

1 Stand with your feet a little wider than hip-width apart and lower yourself into a squat. Put your hands on your knees.

2 Walk forward in this position, bouncing up and down as you go – like a big, heavy toad lumbering across a riverbank. Make a "rivet" sound to go with the movement.

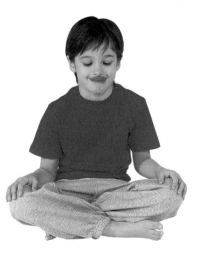

3 When you get tired, sit down on an imaginary log and pretend to catch insects with your tongue. Stick your tongue out as far as it can go, then look toward the tip of your nose and imagine a big, fat fly sitting there (don't strain your eyes though). See if you can catch it with your tongue.

crow walking

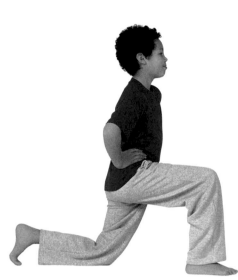

This pose stretches the tops of the quadricep muscles in your thighs and the muscles that run from thigh to pelvis. It also strengthens your buttocks and the backs of your legs.

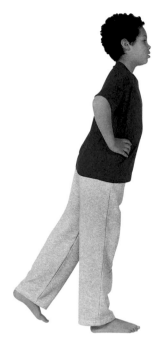

1 Stand with your hands on your hips. Take a big step forward with your right leg. Bend your right leg to a right angle and bring your left knee down to the floor behind you. Pause for a second.

2 Push forward with your left foot and straighten your right leg again, so that you come back up to standing.

3 As you straighten your right leg, take a big step forward with your left leg, bringing it into a right angle. Bring the knee of your right leg down to the floor behind you. Come back up to standing. Keep taking big steps forward in this way. Try to make your movements as smooth and fluid as possible.

👁 Imitate the cawing of a crow as you walk. See if you can make your face look like a crow's.

bunny hops

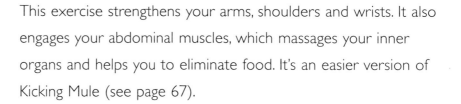

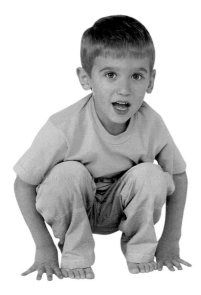

This exercise strengthens your arms, shoulders and wrists. It also engages your abdominal muscles, which massages your inner organs and helps you to eliminate food. It's an easier version of Kicking Mule (see page 67).

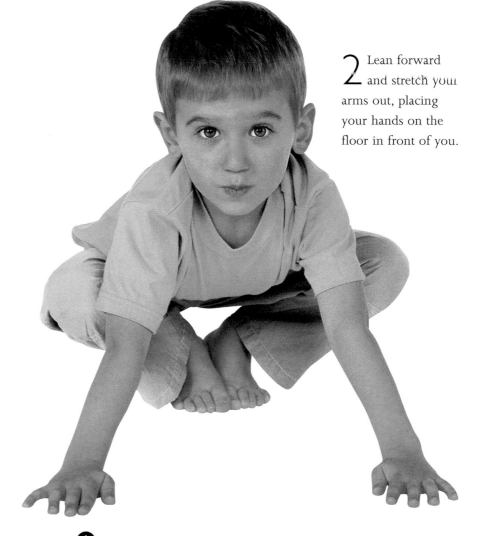

1 Get into a deep squatting position and place your hands on the floor on either side of your feet.

2 Lean forward and stretch your arms out, placing your hands on the floor in front of you.

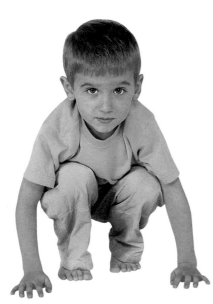

3 Take a hop forward so that your feet land near to or between your hands. Keep repeating this movement.

👁 Pretend that you are a little rabbit hopping around a meadow. You can sing "Run Rabbit Run" if you like.

☺ If you live near rabbits, or have one as a pet, watch how they move their heads and bodies and how they breathe. Can you imitate the facial expressions of a rabbit? What's your favourite thing about a rabbit?

knee walking

This exercise develops your sense of balance and keeps your knee joints healthy. It stretches the quadriceps and psoas muscles on the front of your thighs and hips. It's quite a difficult balancing act, but – whether you manage to do it or not – you can have great fun trying!

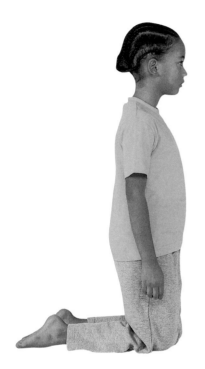

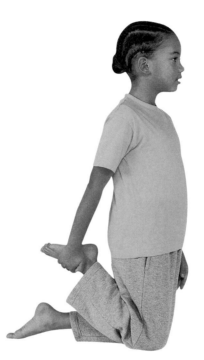

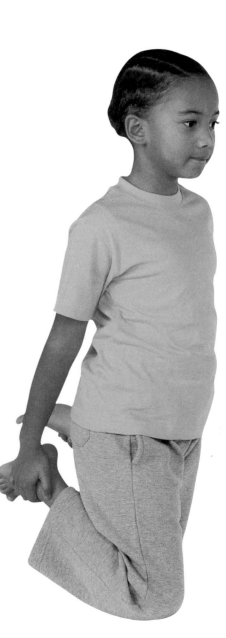

1 Kneel with your knees and feet about hip-distance apart. Let your arms hang loosely by your sides.

This exercise can be hard on your knees so you might want to cover your floor space with folded blankets or mats before you start.

2 Bend your right leg and catch your right foot with your right hand. Bend your left leg and catch your left foot with your left hand so that you are balancing on just your knees. You may find it easier to balance if you focus on a fixed point in front of you.

3 When you've found your balance in this pose try walking around on your knees while holding onto both ankles. Be prepared to fall over a few times though!

swamp monster

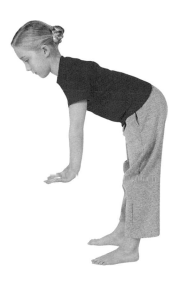

This is a walking version of Standing Sandwich (see pages 44–5). Swamp Monster helps to keep your lower back and the backs of your legs supple. Because you are partly inverted, your brain and the glands in your neck and throat receive a good supply of oxygen-rich blood. This regulates hormonal secretions, which are necessary for the optimum functioning of your body and brain. As a result, you feel totally revitalized.

1 Stand with your feet hip-distance apart and extend forward from your waist, keeping your spine long.

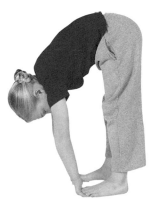

2 Put your hands under your feet with your palms face up.

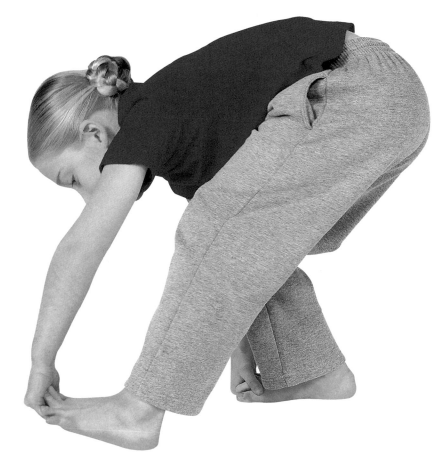

⮂ If you are quite flexible and you want an extra challenge, try keeping your legs straight as you walk. Just for fun, see if you can jump forward with your hands under your feet. Not so easy!

3 Walk forward, stepping your right hand and foot forward first, then your left hand and foot. Pretend that you are a monster crawling out of a swamp.

crab walking

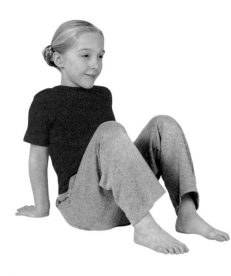

This exercise is an adaptation of a yoga pose known as Table. It keeps your shoulder joints and wrists strong and flexible, strengthens the gluteus muscles around your hips and bottom, and develops your co-ordination and agility.

1 Sit with your legs stretched out in front of you, your hands behind you and your fingers pointing backward. Bend your knees and draw your heels in toward you. Keep your feet flat on the floor.

2 Lift your hips up into the air so that your legs form a right angle and your body looks like a table. You may need to adjust the distance between your hands and feet. Lift up your head and look forward.

3 Take three steps to the right. Now take three steps to the left, back to where you started from. Have fun playing around in the pose – try going forward, backward and turning around in a full circle.

👁 Pretend that you are a crab side-stepping across a beach. What sort of beach are you on? Sandy or stony? How far is it to the sea?

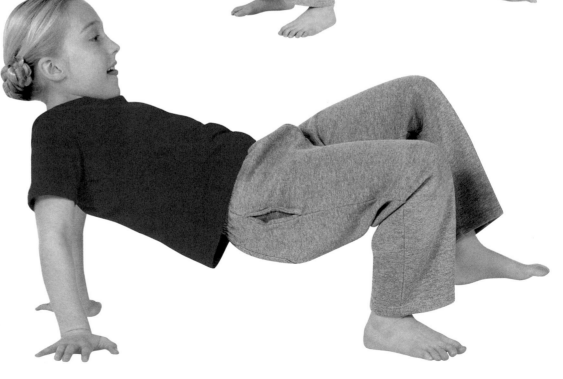

swimming

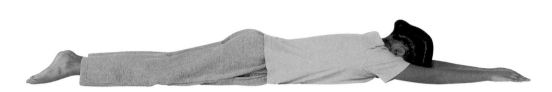

This is a variation of a classical yoga posture known as Locust. Here, because you do the posture dynamically, it looks as though you are doing breast stroke. It is an excellent way of strengthening your back, shoulders, hips and hamstrings.

1 Lie down on your front, with your forehead on the floor and your arms stretched out in front of you.

2 Lift your arms, chest, head and legs off the floor. Slowly bring your arms down to the sides of your body in a swimming movement. At the same time separate your legs.

3 Bend your arms and bring them forward until they point straight ahead of you. At the same time bring your legs together. This requires a fair amount of strength so just do it once at first before releasing the pose and returning to step 1. Gradually, build up the number of times you repeat the movement. Once you're familiar with the exercise, breathe in during step 1, breathe out as your arms go back and breathe in as your arms come forward.

The swimming motion can seem complicated at first. You may need to try it several times before you get it right.

This is quite a strenuous exercise. To make it easier, keep your legs on the floor and just do the upper body movements.

mirror, mirror on the wall

This exercise uses the technique of mirroring and it's an excellent way for adults to lead children through a yoga session. Seeing postures mirrored back to them gives children the visual reference they need to understand how a pose works. Mirroring also builds concentration and co-ordination as well as making children sensitive to the subtle energies of others.

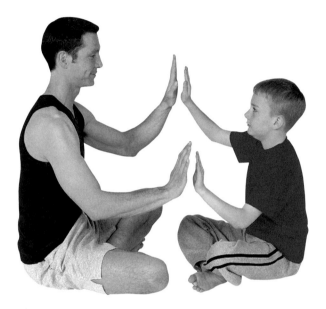

| Sit opposite your child and raise your palms to theirs so that they are close but not touching. Slowly move your hands, getting your child to mirror your movements. Do this for a minute or two and then swap roles.

📖 Encourage your child to feel the heat and energy flowing from your hands to theirs. When you are both sensitized to this energy, close your eyes and rely on the sensations in your palms to guide you. The name for the energy that you feel is *prana* or "life-force".

2 Now get your child to mirror you slowly and silently through a series of postures – try some of the sequences in Chapter 7. When your child is familiar with the poses they can take the lead.

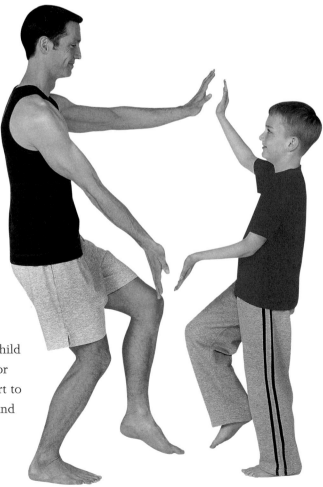

3 Stand opposite your child and ask them to mirror your movements. Now start to dance – make it as weird and wonderful as you like.

asana tag

This is a version of the traditional children's game of "Tag" or "It". The word *asana* means "posture".
Asana Tag makes children familiar with several yoga postures and they have lots of fun in the process.

How to play

You need several people to play *Asana* Tag. One person is "it" and has to "tag" the other players by chasing after and touching them. When someone is tagged they then become "it" and the game starts over. You can avoid being tagged either by running away or by getting into any of these three yoga postures: Tree (see page 49), Eagle (see page 65) or Face-Down Dog (see pages 44–5). To prevent someone staying in a pose for too long, the person who is "it" is allowed to stand three strides away and shout "*maya, maya, maya!*" followed by the name of the person they want to chase. This means that the person in the pose must either run away or quickly get into a new pose.

📖 The word *maya* refers to the web of confusion that people live in before they get to *samadhi* – the place of absolute peace and stillness that is the goal of yoga.

⮀ You can vary this game by adding different postures. If there are enough players, you can include the supported balance on page 99.

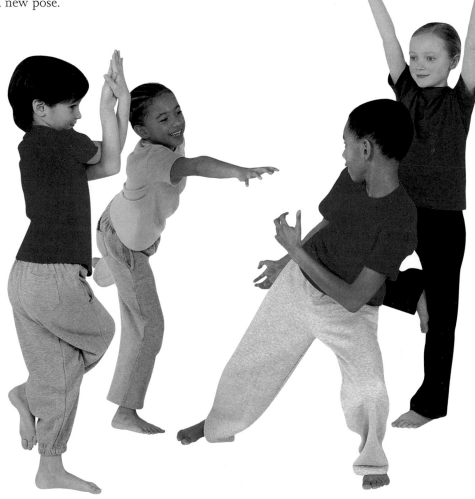

stick in the web

This is the yoga version of the children's game "Stick in the Mud". As well as familiarizing children with several yoga postures, this game is an excellent way of building up co-operation skills.

How to Play

You need at least four people to play Stick in the Web. One person is the *maya* spider (*maya* refers to the web of confusion that we live in; see page 95) and has to catch the other players in their web by chasing and "tagging" them. If a player is caught, they must lie on the ground. They can only be freed by another player crawling underneath them as they do Building a Bridge (see pages 84–5).

You can add variety to this game by introducing other poses. For example, you can free another player by crawling underneath them as they do Face-Down Dog (see pages 44–5) or leap-frogging over them as they bend forward in Standing Sandwich (see pages 44–5) with their hands on their knees.

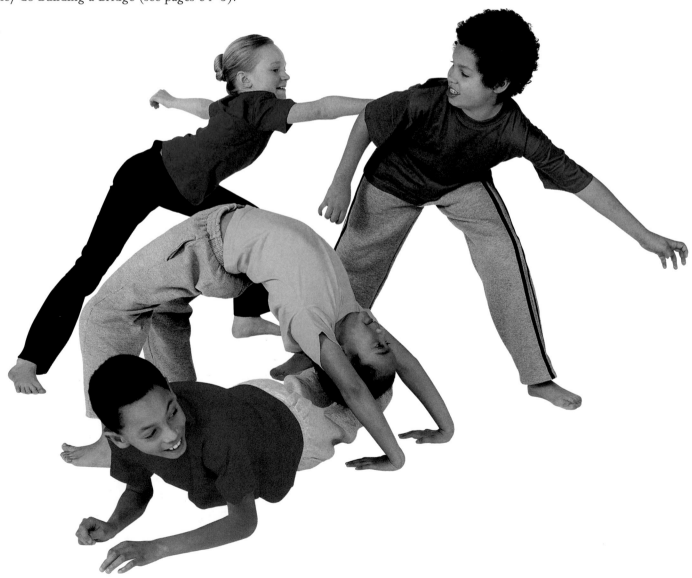

whodunnit yoga

This game develops teamwork and intuition. To play it well, you have to be extremely aware of what is going on around you at all times, and be ready to act immediately. These are the qualities of a good yogi.

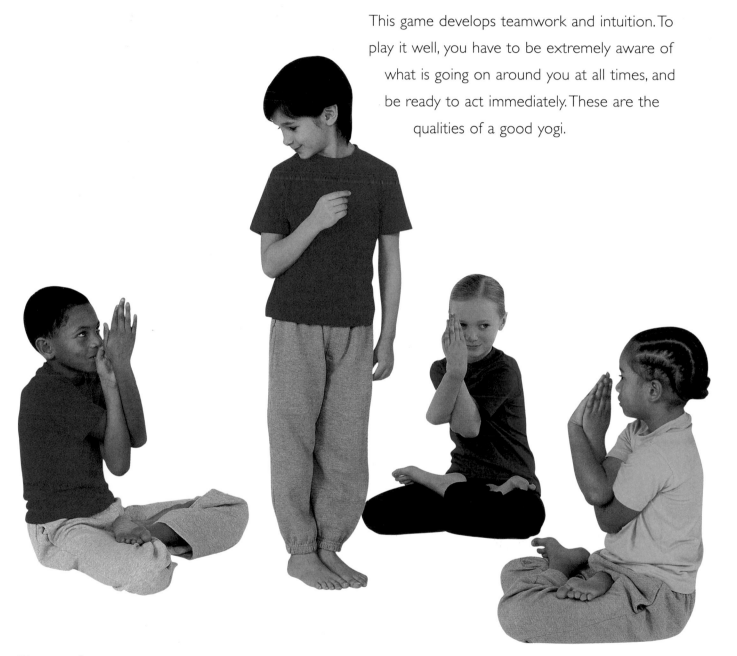

How to play

You need several people to play Whodunnit Yoga (the more players, the more difficult it is). One player, the detective, goes out of the room, while the other players select a ringleader. The ringleader chooses a yoga posture and everyone stands or sits in a circle and adopts that posture.

The detective is called back and stands in the middle of the circle. The ringleader proceeds to change posture at various intervals. The players in the circle must follow suit so fast that the identity of the ringleader remains secret. As soon as the detective spots the ringleader, the game starts over.

asana obstacle race

This is a yoga version of the old sports day race. It is a great way to present a whole sequence of postures to children in a fun and interesting way. When played in a relaxed and non-competitive spirit, it helps kids to develop agility and quick-thinking.

How to play

You need two or more people to play *Asana* Obstacle Race. First, you set up a course with a starting and a finishing line – this is an ideal game to play outside in the summer but you can also do it indoors if you have a big enough space. Divide the course into six or more sections, marking each one with a line, flag or other prop.

Now you're ready to race. Come up to the starting line and squat down like a bunny rabbit. On the count of three, bunny hop (see page 89) forward as fast as you can. When you reach the first line, stop, adopt the first yoga posture (see suggestions below), count backward from ten to zero and then bunny hop on to the next line where you adopt the second yoga position and so on. The first person to reach the finishing line having successfully completed all the postures is the winner.

Decide in advance which yoga postures your race will feature. You could also vary the ways to get from posture to posture, either keeping a single yoga-walk for the whole race, or linking each stage with a different walk. Here are some ideas.

Bunny Hops (see page 89) to ... **STAGE 1: Triangle** (see page 50)	Crab Walking (see page 92) to ... **STAGE 3: Warrior** (see page 53)	Crow Walking (see page 88) to ... **STAGE 5: Eagle** (see page 65)
Walking the Dog (see page 86) to ... **STAGE 2: Half Moon** (see page 51)	Swamp Monster (see page 91) to ... **STAGE 4: Big Butterfly** (see page 73)	Toad Walking (see page 87) to ... **STAGE 6: Tree** (see page 49)

In another version of this game the obstacles consist of people. The course is divided up in the usual way but at the dividing lines you have to either navigate your way past a person in a particular *asana* or do a pose together (see my ideas below). Ideally, you will have about six people playing this variation. It can be played with just two, however, if after each stage, the racer does a yoga walk round a flag or marker and back, to give the "obstacle" player time to change posture.

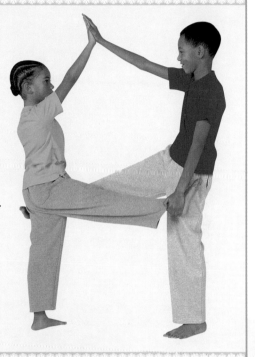

- Building a Bridge (see page 84). Wriggle underneath like a fish.
- Mountain (see page 48). Run around the Mountain three times chirping like a bird.
- Face-Down Dog (see pages 44–5). Scamper underneath like a puppy.
- Triangle (see page 50) and Arrow (see page 52). Do these postures back-to-back.
- Supported balance (see picture opposite). Stand one arm's length apart from your partner. Hold the heel of your partner's right foot in your left hand and get them to hold your right foot in their left hand. Now put your right palm against their left palm and both raise your arms.

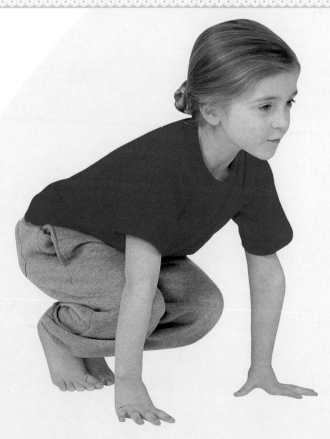

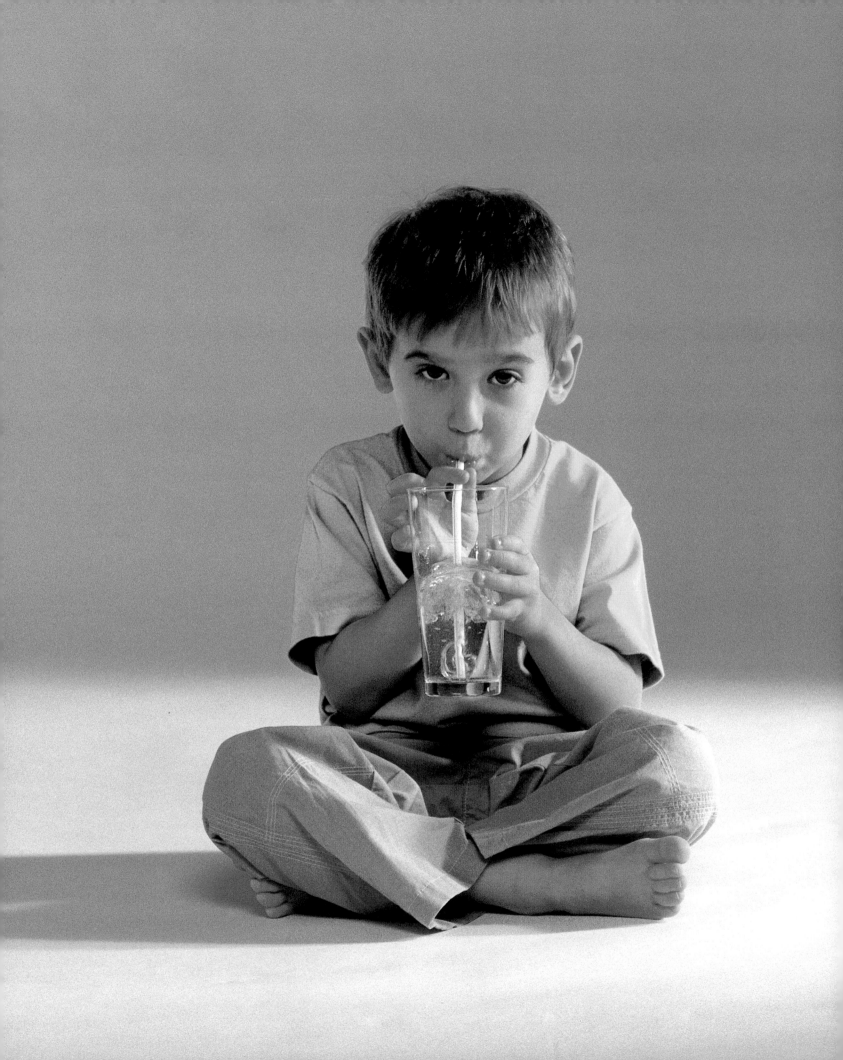

journeying inward

This chapter looks at some of the less physical and more internal aspects of yoga – breathing (or *pranayama*), meditation and deep relaxation.

All of the exercises presented here can help children to gather in their energy, so that it can be used with direction and focus. If we are always "outside" of ourselves, it is difficult not to be dissipated and distracted by our senses. But if we can learn to centre and be still when we need to, we will be able to concentrate more easily on our tasks. In modern society, where we are continually bombarded by stimulation, information and noise, we have lost the habit of simply sitting quietly with ourselves. Yoga offers all of us – both children and adults – a way to come home to ourselves, and to learn to live in peace with who we are, without always running for distraction or entertainment.

what is *pranayama*?

Pranayama is the name given to the breathing techniques that are a central part of yoga. The way that you breathe has a direct effect on your state of mind, your emotions and your behaviour. The better you breathe, the easier you will find it to concentrate, relax and learn. Good breathing also ensures that you have more energy, are less susceptible to tiredness and, when it comes to bedtime, you sleep more deeply. *Pranayama* is the fourth limb of yoga described by Patanjali in one of the most important ancient texts on yoga, the *Yoga Sutras* (see page 18).

Prana – universal energy

Prana, or Chi as it is called in Chinese medicine, is the vital energy of the universe which courses through all living things. It is a kind of subtle electricity, providing vitality and health to our bodies and minds. When *prana* levels are high, we feel vibrant and alive; when they drop below a certain level, we fall ill; and when *prana* leaves the body altogether, we die. That is why it is important to keep our *prana* levels high by eating fresh, healthy food, breathing clean air and practising yoga.

Think about a fresh, green, crunchy stick of celery, full of life and goodness. Now imagine the same stick two weeks later – it's yellow, drooping and soft, and all the goodness has left it. The fresh stick of celery is full of *prana*. The second stick isn't. (This is why live foods, such as sprouted seeds and pulses are so good for us – they transmit their energy into our bodies and keep us healthy.) When we get sick, we become like the old, yellow celery. To get well again, we have to bring more *prana* into our bodies. This idea forms the basis of most Indian, Chinese and Tibetan methods of medicine. *Pranayama* is one way of regulating our levels of *prana* by using the air around us. The most famous text on this subject, the 14th century *Hatha Yoga Pradipika* tells us that "By proper practice of *pranayama* all diseases are eradicated".

Pranayama also has a spiritual purpose: by balancing the energies of the body and the nervous system, it helps to calm and focus the mind so that it becomes receptive to spiritual inspiration. As we become more sensitive to the energy of the universe, we begin to understand our connection with the rest of creation (see page 23). It is thought that many prayers, chants and mantras from the world's religious traditions are specially designed to regulate the breath and open us up to the divine spirit within.

When to start *pranayama*

Children under the age of eight should practise only the first three *pranayama* exercises described on pages 104–5. As a general rule, when you first start to practise yoga, concentrate on giving your child a good grounding in the postures. Then, once they've got to grips with the physical movements, start to encourage them to combine their movements with their breath.

In many of the postures in chapters 2, 3, 4 and 5, I advise you at which point to breathe in and out. Broadly speaking, all upward movements in postures should be accompanied by an in-breath and all downward movements by an out-breath.

One of the simplest postures for teaching your child about synchronizing breath and movement is Albatross (see page 62) in which you raise your arms above your head while breathing in and lower your arms while breathing out. Making the Fire (see page 68) and Mosquito (see page 71) are two other great postures for learning about breath and movement. If your child seems receptive, start to put more emphasis on breathing correctly in all of the yoga postures that they do. If this goes well, they are probably ready to start practising the *pranayama* exercises on the following pages.

If your child doesn't seem receptive to the idea of combining breath and movement, leave this aspect of yoga until they are older. In the meantime, just concentrate on having fun in your posture practice together.

The beauty of breath

If your child has never paid conscious attention to their breathing, start by getting them to do this simple exercise which provides them with a visual reference for their breath. Take a tray of ice cubes straight from the freezer and ask your child to gently blow over the surface. They should see a little cloud – a combination of air and water vapour that comes from their lungs. Explain that the same thing happens when warm breath hits air on a cold day – point this out to them the next time it happens.

If your child seems interested, you could also try explaining the principles of breathing – that when we breathe in air, our lungs absorb oxygen which is pumped by the heart through our arteries and blood vessels to feed every cell in our body. Without this oxygen we cannot survive. The heart then pumps the left-over waste matter – carbon dioxide – back through the veins to the heart and lungs, where it is expelled as we breathe out.

You can also explain the way in which the earth's atmosphere is kept in balance by plants. Whereas we inhale oxygen and exhale carbon dioxide, plants and trees absorb carbon dioxide and give out oxygen – this is why plants and trees are so important and one reason why it is so dangerous to cut down large areas of forest.

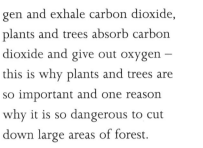

GUIDELINES FOR PRACTISING *PRANAYAMA*

Approach the *pranayama* exercises in this chapter slowly and gently and observe the following guidelines:

- Never strain or make any forceful movements. And don't hold your breath.
- Use the least amount of effort possible in the exercises.

- Stop if you or your child experience any discomfort or shortness of breath.
- Always breathe in and out through your nose (this applies to posture practice as well as to *pranayama*). Nose breathing, as well as lengthening and smoothing your breath, helps to warm and filter air before it reaches your lungs.

pranayama exercises

These exercises offer simple ways to become familiar with the way that you breathe. The first exercise helps you to become aware of the consistency and texture of your breath – for example, whether it is fast or slow, even or ragged. The next two teach you how to make your breathing smooth, regular and balanced by drawing air deeply into your lungs. Techniques such as Up and Down the Mountain and Straw and Bee Breathing teach you how to calm and soothe your mind when you are feeling anxious.

Watching your Breath

Simply observing the way that your breath moves in and out of your body is a spiritual exercise that is practised in many different traditions from Buddhism and Hinduism to Christianity. It is a powerful tool for putting you in touch with your deeper nature (see page 22). It can also have a profound effect on the way that you feel physically and emotionally. Both adults and children become calmer and more "together" after Watching your Breath. The exercise is particularly good for children if they're feeling worried about something. It's great to do immediately before going into a class test or exam. You can do it anywhere and it only takes a few minutes.

Start by sitting quietly and comfortably. Gently breathe in and out through your nose. See how soft you can make your breathing – imagine that you are trying to catch the delicate fragrance of a flower floating by on the breeze. Do this for a minute or so.

Now see if you can tell whether your in-breath is longer than your out-breath or vice-versa? Is one of your nostrils more open than the other? Is the air warmer on the way in to your lungs or on the way out? What is the speed and texture of your breath? Now just observe your breath moving in and out like a wave. Do this for a few minutes.

Wave Breathing

This breathing technique is also known as diaphragmatic breathing because it uses your diaphragm alone to draw air into your body. Your diaphragm is a large dome-shaped sheet of muscle that lies at the bottom of your ribcage. As you breathe in, the dome flattens out, pushing your abdominal organs down and forward and making your belly swell outward (which is why this type of breathing is sometimes called abdominal breathing). Then, as you breathe out, your diaphragm muscle relaxes back into its dome shape and your belly becomes flat again.

To practise Wave Breathing, lie down on your back in *Shavasana* (see page 32) and put your right hand on your

Place a small, light object, such as a rubber duck or a paper boat, on your belly and see if you can make it move by drawing air deeply into your lungs so that your belly swells outward – this is Wave Breathing.

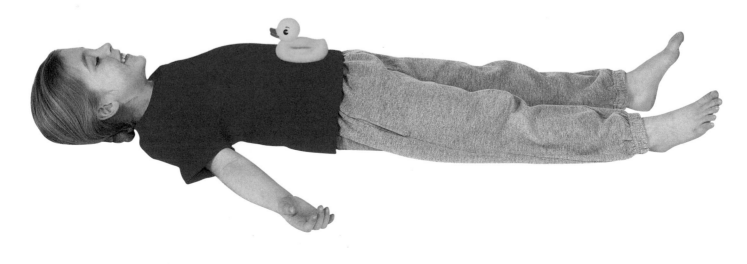

Balloon Breathing teaches you to use your diaphragm to breathe deeply and fully. The secret of the technique is to imagine that you really do have a balloon inflating and deflating inside your belly.

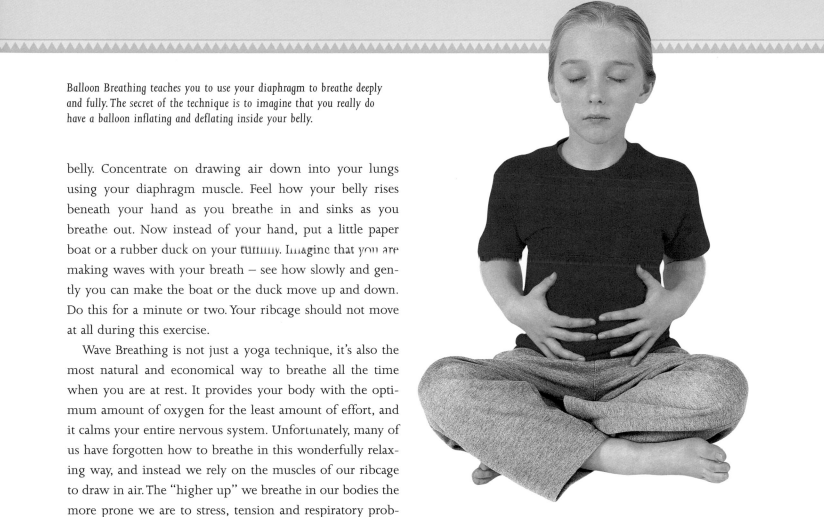

belly. Concentrate on drawing air down into your lungs using your diaphragm muscle. Feel how your belly rises beneath your hand as you breathe in and sinks as you breathe out. Now instead of your hand, put a little paper boat or a rubber duck on your tummy. Imagine that you are making waves with your breath – see how slowly and gently you can make the boat or the duck move up and down. Do this for a minute or two. Your ribcage should not move at all during this exercise.

Wave Breathing is not just a yoga technique, it's also the most natural and economical way to breathe all the time when you are at rest. It provides your body with the optimum amount of oxygen for the least amount of effort, and it calms your entire nervous system. Unfortunately, many of us have forgotten how to breathe in this wonderfully relaxing way, and instead we rely on the muscles of our ribcage to draw in air. The "higher up" we breathe in our bodies the more prone we are to stress, tension and respiratory problems. This is why stressed people look as though they have their shoulders hunched up around their ears. Making sure that you breathe diaphragmatically will have both an immediate and a long-term effect on your health and wellbeing, so start right now!

Balloon Breathing

Another way of learning – or relearning – to breathe diaphragmatically is to practise Balloon Breathing. Sit up straight in a cross-legged position, breathe out and, at the moment when your lungs are empty, put both hands on your belly so that the ends of your middle fingers touch over your belly button. Now, as you breathe in, imagine that your belly is a balloon that is slowly filling up with air. As your belly swells outward, notice how your middle fingers move apart from each other. Now breathe out

and imagine the balloon deflating – watch your fingers come back together again. Try this a few more times. When you are accustomed to breathing in this way, try to do it all the time you are at rest.

Up and Down the Mountain

This *pranayama* exercise is also known as "alternate nostril breathing". In yoga it is believed that life energy, or *prana* (see page 102), travels around our body through hundreds of invisible passageways called *nadis* and that, by breathing alternately through each nostril, we can keep these passageways unblocked. This, in turn, keeps us healthy and maintains a good balance between body and mind. From a scientific perspective, alternate nostril breathing can help to bring the right and left sides of the brain into balance. It has been extremely beneficial in the treatment of children with

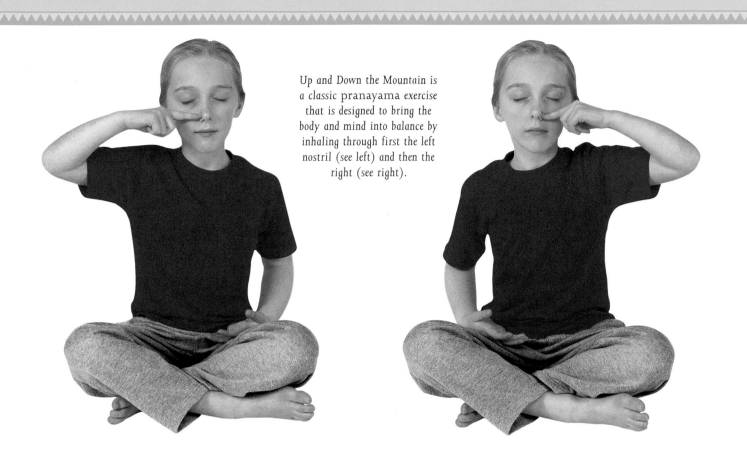

Up and Down the Mountain is a classic pranayama *exercise that is designed to bring the body and mind into balance by inhaling through first the left nostril (see left) and then the right (see right).*

attention deficit disorder (ADD) and attention deficit hyperactivity disorder (ADHD). It can calm you if you're feeling agitated and refresh you if you're feeling sluggish.

Start by sitting comfortably with your spine straight. Spend a few moments letting your breathing become calm and regular. Now imagine that your nose is a mountain: the space between your eyebrows is the top of the mountain, and the place where your nostrils meet your face is the bottom of the mountain.

Imagine that your house is at the bottom of the mountain, just by your left nostril. To collect your eggs for breakfast you have to travel all the way to the top of the mountain and then down the other side to where the egg seller lives, just by your right nostril. Then, once you've collected your eggs, you have to travel all the way to the top of the mountain again and back down to your house. Luckily, you have a special chairlift to take you there and back – your own breath.

Start the exercise by breathing out completely and then blocking off your right nostril with the index finger of your right hand. Breathe in slowly and softly through your left nostril. When your lungs are full you have reached the top of the mountain.

Now release your right hand and use the index finger of your left hand to block off your left nostril. Slowly and softly breathe out through your right nostril to get to the bottom of the mountain and collect your eggs.

It's time to go back up the mountain with your eggs. Keep your left-hand index finger in place as you breathe in through your right nostril. When your lungs are full, you are at the top of the mountain. Now release your left hand and once more block off your right nostril using your right index finger. Breathe out slowly and softly through your left nostril to return home. Repeat the entire trip three times and then lie down and rest. Remember that mountain air can be very tiring, so don't overdo it!

Straw Breathing

This *pranayama* exercise focuses on lengthening your exhalation, which has a soothing and calming effect on your nervous system. Straw Breathing is great for children because they can immediately see the effects of their lungs emptying. Straw Breathing is particularly recommended for asthma sufferers as it helps them to expel carbon dioxide effectively from their bodies (an inability to exhale fully is a defining symptom of asthma).

Take a glass of water or juice and put a straw in it. Sit up straight and breathe in deeply. Now, as you breathe out, blow slowly through the straw to create a stream of bubbles. Keep the bubbles going for the length of your out-breath and try to make them as even and regular as you can. When your lungs are empty, take the straw out of your mouth, breathe in and then repeat the exercise. Do this a few times, but don't over-exert yourself.

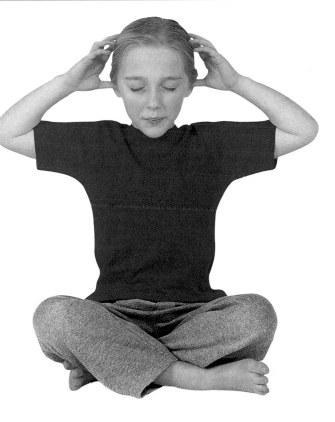

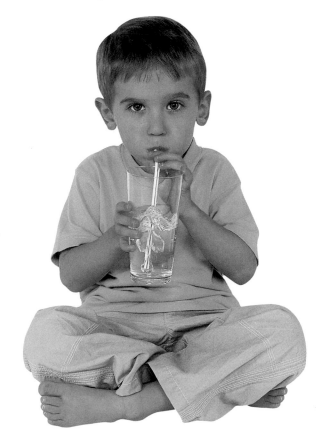

Straw Breathing (below left) and Bee Breath (above) bring your awareness to the way in which you breathe out. Both techniques encourage you to make your exhalations long and smooth and this has an immediate soothing effect on your entire nervous system.

Bee Breath

Like Straw Breathing, Bee Breath also focuses your attention on and lengthens your out-breath. It is very effective for soothing children who are feeling stressed or over-tired. It's also good when children are having trouble sleeping.

Sit or lie in a comfortable position and lightly block off your ears with your thumbs. Rest your fingers on top of your head and close your eyes. Take a deep breath in and, as you breathe out, hum like a bee. Keep the sound steady until your lungs are empty. Now breathe in and do it again. When you're used to the exercise, try experimenting with it. Where do you feel the vibration of the humming sound? What happens if you make the note higher or lower? Can you feel the vibration moving up or down your body?

what is meditation?

Meditation is about cultivating inner silence and stillness – about noticing what is going on around you without reacting to it. Finding the still and silent core within yourself makes you less likely to be distracted, upset or bowled over by events that happen to you in your daily life. Practised regularly and over time, meditation puts you in touch with the deepest parts of yourself, beyond the chatter of everyday thoughts and feelings. Meditation grounds you in your "big self" (see pages 22–3), which is the source of strength and happiness in life.

As well as finding a place of stillness, meditation is also about learning to see clearly. We usually paint the world around us with our likes and dislikes, our assumptions and prejudices and, as a result, we don't see situations as they really are. This is called projection. Meditation is about withdrawing our projections so that we can see things as they really are, and respond to them appropriately.

Meditation is a state of pure awareness. We can get a sense of this by practising the meditation or awareness exercises on the following pages: awareness of our surroundings, our breath, our body and our thoughts and emotions. As this awareness broadens, we also become aware that we are aware, and in very advanced stages of meditation, we start to pass beyond the confines of our identity. It is then that we begin to realize our unity with the world around us; in other words, we are the ocean and not the wave (see pages 22–3).

One traditional image for the stages of meditation is the lotus flower. The lotus takes root in mud at the bottom of a

The lotus flower symbolizes our ability to grow out of delusion and realize our full potential through the practice of meditation. The flower, which opens on the surface of the water, represents the blossoming of our "big self" – that part of us which is pure and divine.

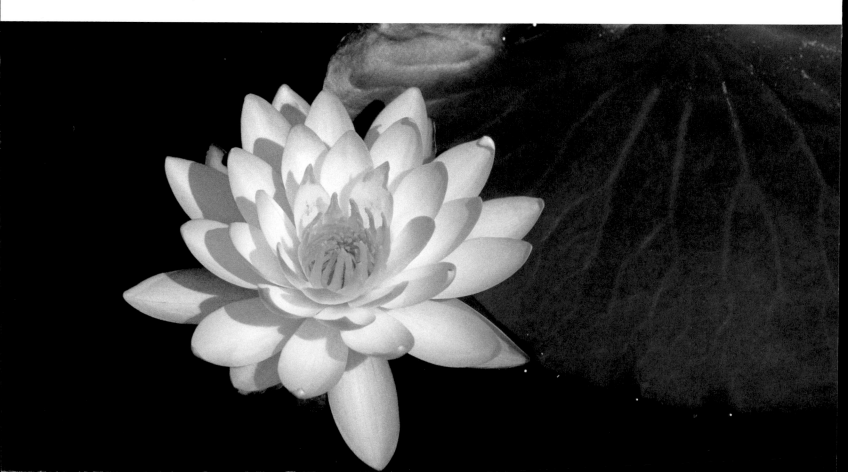

GUIDELINES FOR PRACTISING MEDITATION

- Introduce meditation little by little. Rather than deciding that from now on it will be a formal part of your yoga practice together, just take it gradually and see how your child responds.

- There are two types of exercise on pages 110–13; those that concentrate on tuning in to your surroundings (Video Camera Head and Yellow Submarine) and those that focus on your inner world (Balloons, Chasing Away the Clouds and Love, Love, Love). Always start with the first type of meditation.

- Most children are extremely suggestible and are able to enter a meditative and relaxed state deeply and quickly. For this reason, it's important to keep the exercises short, and to bring children back into the world of the senses through reassuring touches, words and smiles.

- Don't make children close their eyes during meditation if they don't want to. It can make some children nervous. Besides, in some traditions, such as Tibetan Buddhism, meditation is usually taught with the eyes open so that the meditator can keep a strong connection with the outer world, and blend their practice with the rest of their life.

- Read through the exercises on the following pages and try practising them yourself (they're just as good for adults as they are for kids). Then, when you feel you understand them, guide your child through them, explaining the principles in age-appropriate language.

- Some people have a more visual imagination than others, so don't worry if you or your child find some of the visualization exercises difficult. It is more important to feel the object or the situation than to actually see it.

- If you want to include meditation in your morning yoga session, it's best to meditate first and do your posture practice afterward. If, however, you're practising in the evening, do your posture practice first and meditate afterward. This way the day starts quietly and builds up into activity, and ends by winding down from activity into stillness.

lake, representing our delusion and lack of clear vision. As our consciousness is gradually awakened through meditation, the plant reaches up through the water, and finally a beautiful flower blooms on the surface of the lake.

The problem of defining meditation

It is misleading to think that meditation is something that can be achieved by effort or by following a series of steps. True meditation is a simple, natural state in which there is no goal to be strived for and no exercise to do. What we call meditation is really a way of preparing the mind for stillness.

It's a bit like cleaning your house in readiness for a potential visitor: all you can do is prepare, because you're not sure when the visitor will arrive or what they will look like.

When to start meditation

It's usually advisable to wait until your child is eight-years-old or over before you start meditation practice, but you will be the best judge of when your child is receptive. As a general rule, wait until your child has a strong sense of personal identity and of the world around them before you begin to explore the realms of inner space.

meditation exercises

These exercises start with the observation of your outer environment and gradually move on to your inner environment. The "outer" exercises help to hone your concentration and your awareness of your surroundings. The "inner" exercises teach you ways to deal with distracting thoughts or negative feelings, and how to cultivate positive emotions such as love.

Video Camera Head

This beautifully simple meditation game was developed by Valentino Giacomin at the Alice Project in India (see page 10). You can play Video Camera Head anywhere, but it is especially good in places of natural beauty. For the "play back" part of the exercise, you need either a partner or a pen and a piece of paper.

Sit in a comfortable position and imagine that you have a video camera in the place that your head normally occupies. Now quietly start to "film" whatever you can see in front of you. Remember that a video camera doesn't think about what it sees, it's just there to record things. So, for example, if you see a tree, don't start thinking about whether it is a pretty tree or an ugly tree or whether you'd like to climb it, just film it – nothing else. Try to see everything as if for the first time. Even if you see someone you know, don't get distracted by your thoughts and feelings about them. Just record their actions.

Do this for a minute or two. When you become more familiar with the exercise, you can do it for longer periods. Then turn around so that you are facing in the opposite direction and "play back" what you just filmed by telling your yoga partner all the different things you saw. Alternatively, you can write down everything that you saw on a piece of paper.

As you get better at Video Camera Head, examine things in greater detail. For example, notice each blade of grass, each fibre in the carpet or the tiny pores on a person's skin. There is an infinite wealth of detail in everything around you – all you have to do is look. As a variation of this exercise, you can play the memory game in which you arrange random items on a tray which you then show to a group of players for up to one minute. The players have to see how many of the items they can "record" and remember.

Yellow Submarine

This exercise is similar to Video Camera Head, except that here you become "all ears" instead of "all eyes". You'll be amazed at how many different noises are going on all around you – and even inside you – and how good you become at listening.

Cup your hands over your eyes and imagine that you are inside a big yellow submarine. Like submarines, which rely upon sonar, the only way that you can receive information about the outside world is through the medium of sound. And like sonar, which simply registers sound on a screen, your job is to record sound without thinking about it. Don't respond to different noises by categorizing them as pleasant or unpleasant – just let them enter your head without comment. For the next two stages of Yellow Submarine you will need a partner.

Get your partner to put on a song or piece of music (it could be "Yellow Submarine" by *The Beatles*!). Now turn on your sonar and let the sound flow into you. In a second your partner is going to turn down the volume of the music so that it is barely audible – your job is to keep focusing on the sound no matter how faint it becomes. A variation of this is for your partner to play a series of tunes at very low volume. This is followed by a "play back" session in which you name the tunes that you heard.

For stage two, you simply sit still in a comfortable position. You can close your eyes if you want to. Turn on your sonar and listen to the sounds coming from inside the room (for example, your partner is going to make some sounds of their own by rustling paper or clicking a pen). How many different sounds can you hear? Now extend the range of your sonar to beyond the room. What sounds are coming to your ear from outside? Don't get carried away by the sounds and by your thoughts about them. Don't dwell upon whether the sounds are pleasant or annoying – just let them come and go. What is the most distant or the faintest sound you can hear?

In the final stage of Yellow Submarine, you turn your sonar in upon yourself and listen to your own breath. You will need to be as quiet and still as you can – if you can't quite hear your breath, breathe more heavily so that you can hear the air travelling through your nose. Then gradually make your breath soft again and see if you can keep in touch with the sound. Now try to follow the rhythm of your breath as it flows in and out, coming and going like waves rolling on a beach.

Balloons

This meditation exercise teaches you that you don't have to get tangled up in your thoughts and emotions. You can let go of them whenever you want to, just like letting go of a balloon and watching it float away.

Imagine a huge blue sky in front, behind, above and below you (you might find this easier if you close your eyes). This is the infinite sky inside you. In yoga it is called the "heart-mind" and it is always peaceful and pure. Take a few moments to relax deeply into this space. Allow yourself to feel perfectly safe and at home.

Imagine that your thoughts and feelings are like balloons floating through this clear blue sky. When you sense one floating by, catch its string and hold it for a few moments.

It's wonderful to practise meditation exercises such as Video Camera Head outdoors in beautiful surroundings. Meditation can help to intensify your appreciation of beauty – rather than getting caught up in an internal dialogue about what's in front of you, you become able to see in a much more pure way.

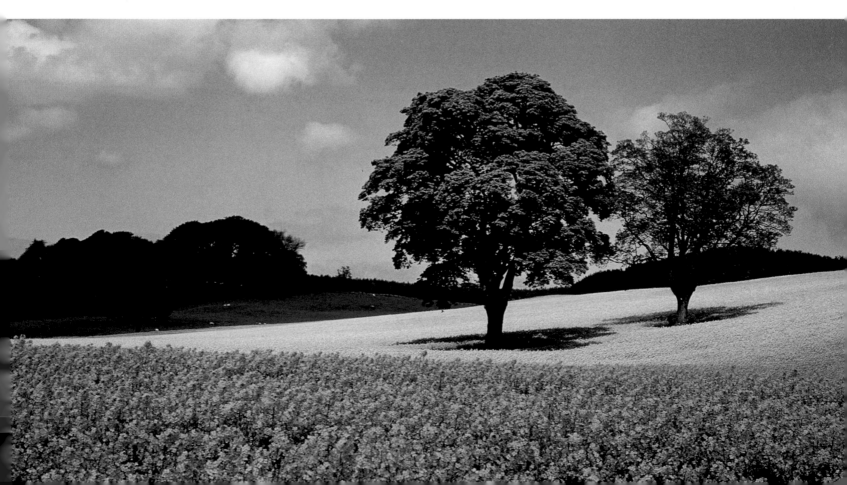

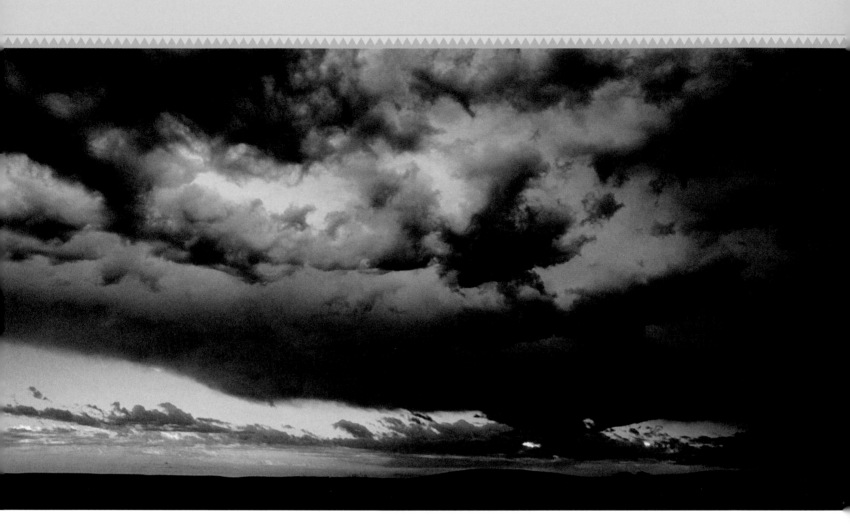

How big is it? What colour is it? Is it bright or dull? Perhaps there is a picture or some words on it? What shape is it? It doesn't have to be round – it could be square or triangular, or it might be one of those long, thin balloons that you can twist into any shape you like. Does the balloon tug fiercely at the string or is it gently floating? How does it make you feel to be near it?

When you've had a good look at the balloon, let go of the string and allow it to float away across the sky. With each breath you take, the balloon wafts further away until it disappears from your awareness. Now wait peacefully for the next thought-balloon to come along.

If you prefer, instead of letting the balloon float away, you can stick an imaginary pin in it. Don't do this if you find it jarring though.

Clouds are an excellent visual symbol for negative or destructive emotions. As with feelings of anger, resentment or anxiety, clouds are transient things that form and disperse without causing any damage.

Chasing Away the Clouds

This exercise is similar to Balloons in that it helps you to free yourself from any negative feelings such as doubt, worry, anger, sadness and fear. Take some time to practise Chasing Away the Clouds whenever you are feeling troubled or "clouded over".

Imagine a huge blue sky in front, behind, above and below you, just like you did in the previous exercise (again, you might find this easier if you close your eyes). Remember that this place is always peaceful and, because it's inside you, you can return to it at any time.

Picture any negative feelings as clouds passing across your sky. Sit quietly and look at these clouds for a while – observe their shapes, colours and textures. Perhaps they have shapes or faces in them? Perhaps they change as you look at them? Get to know them really well and even be friendly toward them. Remember that, no matter how big and dark the clouds that pass across it, the sky never gets damaged. In the same way, strong feelings such as doubt, anger, sadness and fear cannot hurt us.

When you feel ready to let your "thought-clouds" go, say "goodbye" and imagine them dispersing and disappearing each time you breathe out. Gradually, your sky becomes bright and blue again and you feel well, happy and free of negative emotions.

Love, Love, Love

This meditation focuses on love, the most important of all human emotions. Love plays a central role in all the great spiritual traditions, including yoga, where it holds the key to realizing our full potential. Through love we can break through our feelings of self-centredness and loneliness and come to know who we really are.

Practising Love, Love, Love is a great way to beat the blues and build self-esteem. When you love yourself unconditionally, there is no room left for negativity. And extending love to others has an incredibly positive effect on all your relationships. It enables you to go out without fear or shyness, and be warm and friendly to everyone around you. As a result, people respond warmly and positively to you.

There are five parts to this meditation. Find out which ones work best for you and focus on these. Stage one is called "out with the bad, in with the good" and it's good for when you are feeling sad, angry or frustrated. Sit down, get quiet and comfortable and do the Checking In exercise on page 30. Now visualize any negative feelings as grimy black smoke. Try to imagine where this smoke is located inside your body and, every time you exhale, picture the smoke leaving your body and disappearing into space.

When all the smoke has gone, imagine that you are breathing in love in the form of bright white light. Each inhalation suffuses your body with light and you feel full of love and joy. Do this until you feel filled to the brim with loving energy.

Stage two is called "finding the source" and you'll need a partner. Sit down quietly and gaze at each other. Make your body as relaxed as you can and concentrate on really looking deeply into your partner's eyes. You may find that you feel like smiling or laughing – that's fine, but whatever happens, don't break eye contact.

Now try to connect with the space of love and kindness that lies deep within you. To make this easier, you may like to think back to a time when you felt intense love or friendship, either for the person in front of you or someone else, maybe even a pet. Keep hold of that feeling and let it grow until it fills you.

Continue to sit with your partner for stage three. Imagine that you have a glittering diamond inside your chest where your heart is – this is your source of infinite love. As you relax, the diamond starts growing and growing until your whole body is glittering with love. Imagine that you can emit rays of light from your "heart-diamond" so that your partner becomes filled with love too. Keep looking at your partner and say "I love you".

The fourth part of Love, Love, Love consists of sending out rays of loving light to other people who are not in the room. This could be your family, friends and even people you don't know; for example, people living in difficult conditions in other countries. Visualize your love flying out to them at the speed of light and making them feel happy.

The fifth and final stage involves sending out love to those people you don't really like or have problems with. This is the biggest challenge of all – if you find it hard, come back for a moment to all those feelings of love that you experienced in the previous stages of this meditation. If you persevere with this final stage, it often improves your relationship with the person concerned.

the sleeping yogi

This is a deep relaxation exercise that can restore flagging energy levels and help your child to unwind in times of stress or to recuperate after illness. You can also practise the Sleeping Yogi as part of your daily yoga routine to keep your child relaxed and centred. Although it's called the Sleeping Yogi, your child stays awake for the duration of the exercise.

If you are guiding your child through Sleeping Yogi for the first time, keep it brief – a couple of minutes is enough. Children can go into deep relaxation very quickly. Later you can make it longer by going into more detail and extending the visualizations. Talk your child through the exercise at all times – your voice provides a link back to the waking state. Bring your child out of relaxation slowly and gradually so that they don't get disorientated.

1 Ask your child to lie down on the floor in *Shavasana* or *Shavasana* Sandwich (see pages 32–3). Put a blanket over them if it's cold and tell them to get really comfortable. Ask your child to imagine that their body is melting into the floor like chocolate on a hot day. They should relax all their muscles and focus on the contact between their body and the floor. Encourage them to listen to any sounds coming from inside the room and then from outside the room.

2 The next part of the Sleeping Yogi is called "sailing through the body". You are going to name each part of your child's body and, as you do so, ask them to try to imagine that a tiny boat is sailing to that part of them. Tell them to bring all their attention to that part of their body and have a really good look at it with their inner eye.

Here's the route that the boat should take. Read this list aloud (after you name each body part, remember to take a pause to allow the boat to complete its journey).

"Your right hand and fingers. The lower part of your right arm. Your upper arm. The right side of your chest. The right side of your tummy. Your right thigh. Your right knee. Your right shin. Your right foot. The whole of the right side of your body."

Now name all the same body parts, but on the left side of your child's body. Finally, tell the sleeping yogi to imagine the boat sailing to both arms, then both legs, then to their chest, tummy and back, and then up to their neck and head.

3 Now it's time to do a short visualization. Guide your child through Balloons (see page 111) or Love, Love, Love (see page 113). Alternatively, you can make up your own visualization that features a beautiful landscape such as a forest or a waterfall. If you like, you can read aloud the following visualization to your child.

"Imagine that you are lying on a bed of soft, warm moss. You feel very relaxed and comfortable. A gentle, warm rain starts to fall on your body. It washes away your feelings of tiredness, worry, sadness and anger – all the things that make you feel bad. Now the sun is coming out and bringing with it a beautiful, multicoloured rainbow. Coloured light pours down from this rainbow and fills

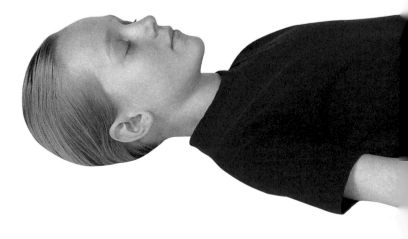

THE GUARDIAN ANGEL

An alternative to the visualization part of the Sleeping Yogi (step 3) is an exercise called the Guardian Angel. Explain to your child that everyone has a guardian angel, whose job it is to love them and keep them safe and sound. A guardian angel can be called upon at any time of the day or night and he or she is always kind and smiling. Children can visualize guardian angels in whatever way they like – as a character from a book or television, a familiar friend or someone completely made-up. Children who have trouble falling asleep may find it helpful to visualize their guardian angel last thing at night.

your body with every colour you can imagine. With this light comes happiness, health, confidence and joy. Immerse yourself in these wonderful feelings."

4 Now it's time to return to the outside world. Guide your child back using these instructions. "Slowly tune in to the sounds you can hear from inside the room … and now the sounds you can hear from outside the room. Focus on the feeling of your body in contact with the floor. When you're ready, slowly start to move your fingers, toes, wrists and ankles. Gently roll your head from side to side. Stretch your arms above your head and give your spine a long stretch. Hug your knees into your chest and gently roll from side to side. Now roll onto your right side and lay your head on your arm. When you feel like it, come slowly up to sitting."

After the Sleeping Yogi, children can feel very creative. Have some paper and pens or crayons ready and encourage them to write or to draw whatever comes into their head.

You can ensure that your child has a deep and restful sleep by doing the Sleeping Yogi at bedtime. The sequence is exactly the same, except that instead of doing the final stage, you gently encourage them to fall asleep by stroking their head.

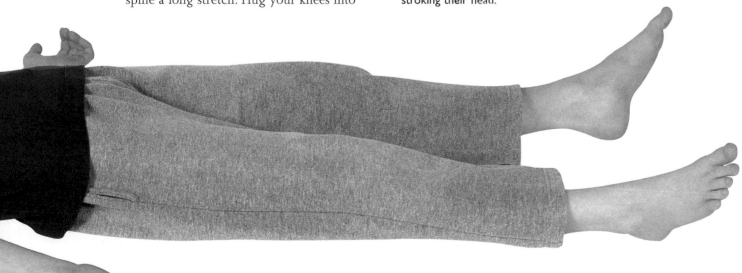

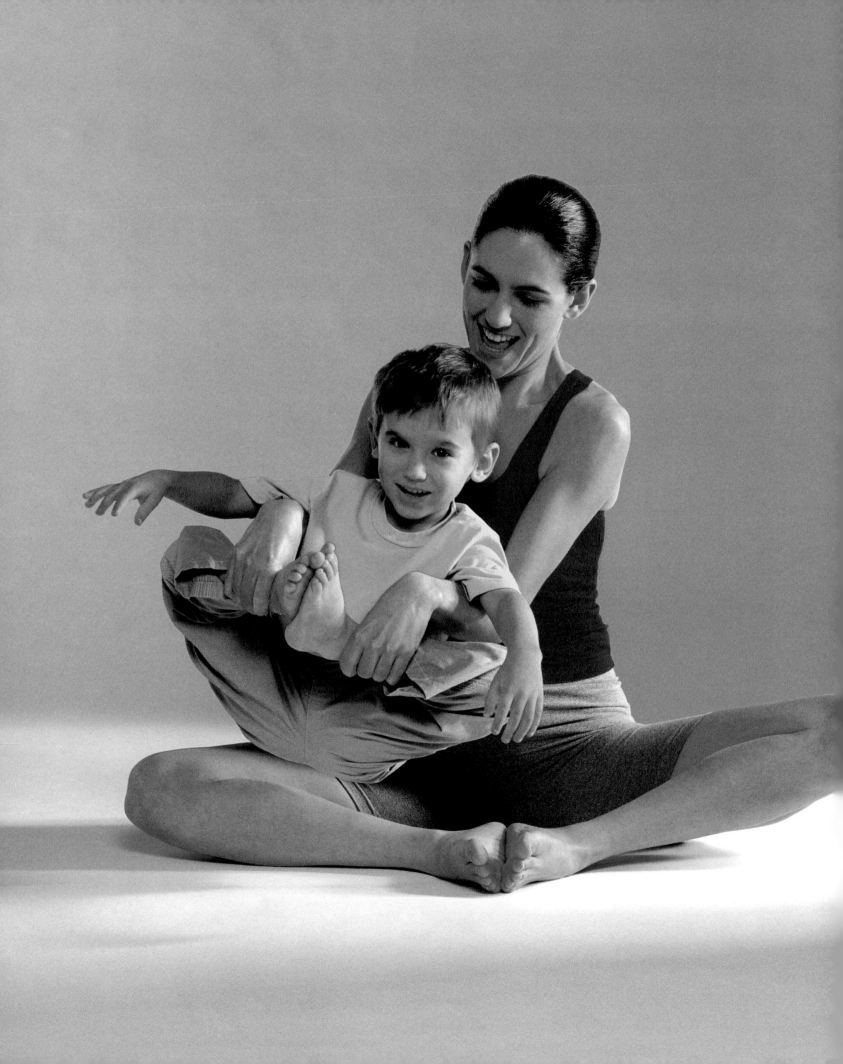

putting it all together

In this chapter I've suggested four sequences made up of various postures and techniques from other chapters. Each sequence forms a self-contained yoga practice. I've designed the first sequence to wake you up when you're feeling sluggish and the second to calm you down when you're buzzing with nervous energy. The third sequence will perk you up if you're feeling under the weather, and the fourth sequence is an imaginative voyage in which you create your own fantastic adventure.

At the heart of doing yoga with kids is the ability to invent and improvise. So don't just follow my ideas for sequences – make up your own too. Be adventurous and try out new things – it's all too easy to stick with familiar postures. Always warm up first (see Chapter 2) and consider including at least one breath or meditation exercise (see Chapter 6). The guidelines on page 47 will help you to combine the main posture-types that you need for a balanced practice.

wake me up

This is a dynamic, stimulating sequence for when you are feeling dull or sluggish. It really helps to counteract lethargy and inertia. A nice way to begin is with a minute of OM chanting (see page 31), followed by Shaking it Up (see page 38), gently at first, then a little more vigorously. Do a few fairly

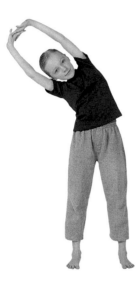

1. WINDY TREE

(page 39)

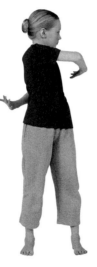

2. HELICOPTER

(page 40)

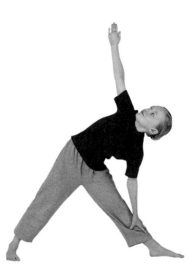

3. TRIANGLE

(page 50)

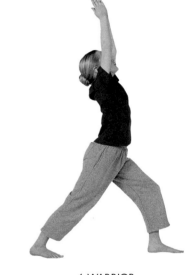

4. WARRIOR

(page 53)

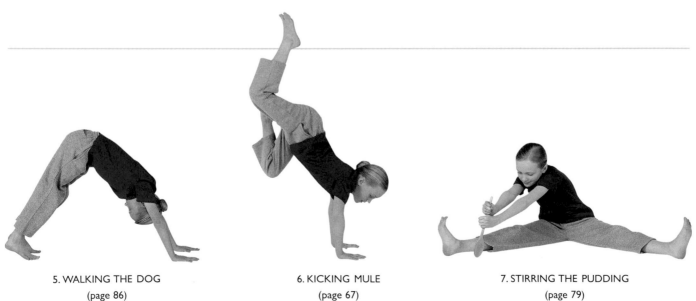

5. WALKING THE DOG

(page 86)

6. KICKING MULE

(page 67)

7. STIRRING THE PUDDING

(page 79)

quick rounds of Greeting the Sun (see pages 44–5) and then begin the sequence. Relax at the end by doing some Wave Breathing (see page 104) in *Shavasana* (see page 32). By the way, don't confuse lethargy with genuine tiredness – if you're suffering from fatigue, do the sequence on page 122.

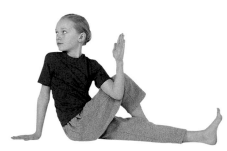

8. SAILING BOAT

(page 56)

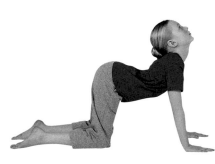

9. CAT

(page 69)

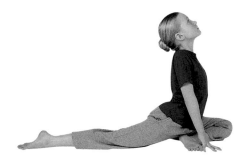

10. PIGEON KING, STEP 2

(page 64)

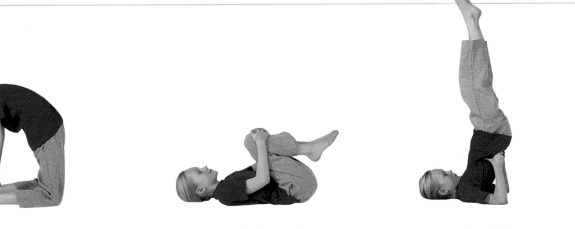

11. CAMEL

(page 57)

12. ROCKING THE BOAT

(page 34)

13. ROCKET

(page 58)

calm me down

This sequence helps you to focus when you're feeling hyper or anxious. The sequence starts dynamically then gradually becomes quieter and more restful. Start off with three to five rounds of Greeting the Sun (see pages 44–5) – do each stage slowly and with real control. Rest in *Shavasana* (see page 32) for a

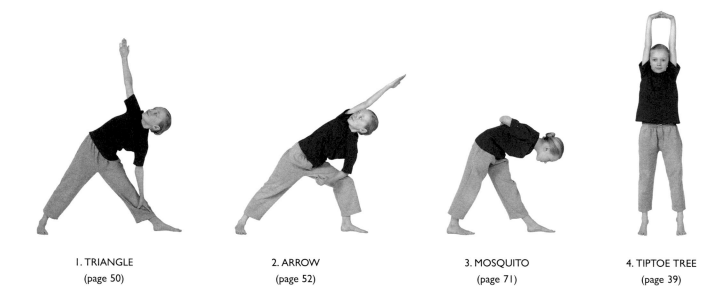

1. TRIANGLE
(page 50)

2. ARROW
(page 52)

3. MOSQUITO
(page 71)

4. TIPTOE TREE
(page 39)

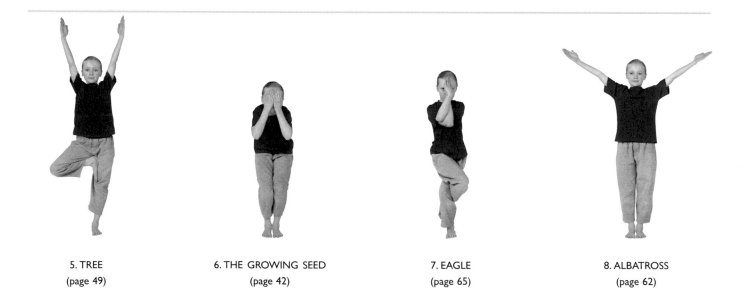

5. TREE
(page 49)

6. THE GROWING SEED
(page 42)

7. EAGLE
(page 65)

8. ALBATROSS
(page 62)

minute or two after Greeting the Sun, and again after the standing poses. Finish the sequence with the Sleeping Yogi relaxation (see pages 114–15). To extend the whole sequence, start off with Puppet (see page 41) and Chopping the Wood (see page 80). Both postures are great for releasing nervous energy.

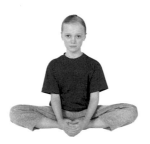

9. LITTLE BUTTERFLY, STEP 1
(page 72)

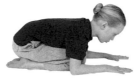

10. MOUSE AND MAKING THE FIRE (page 68)

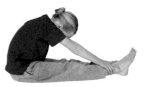

11. SITTING SANDWICH (SLOWLY) (page 54)

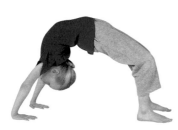

12. BUILDING A BRIDGE
(pages 84–5)

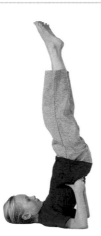

13. ROCKET
(page 58)

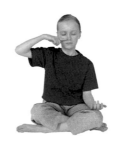

14. UP AND DOWN THE MOUNTAIN
(page 106)

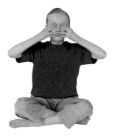

15. BEE BREATH WITH CLOSING THE DOORS
(page 107 and page 131)

pick me up

If you are feeling weak or recovering from an illness, you will need to keep your yoga practice soft and gentle. Your aim should be to nourish and heal, rather than to tire yourself out. The following restorative sequence will help to relieve fatigue and weakness and to shift stagnant energy in your body without taxing your already depleted system. If any of the postures feel too demanding, just leave them out. Start by lying down in *Shavasana* (see page 32) and observing your breath for a few minutes. While you are lying down you could also try visualizing your feelings of tiredness or illness as clouds that are dispersing and disappearing (see page 112). End the sequence by relaxing in the Sleeping Yogi (see pages 114–5).

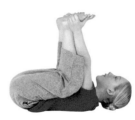

I. ROCKING THE BOAT

(page 34)

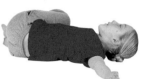

2. DEAD BUG

(page 34)

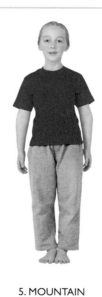

3. ROLLING TWIST

(page 35)

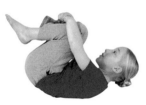

4. DYNAMIC EASY BRIDGE

(page 36)

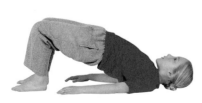

5. MOUNTAIN

(page 48)

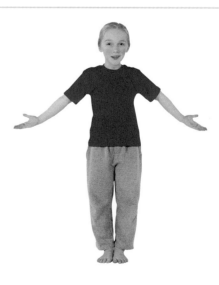

6. ALBATROSS

(page 62)

At the end of the sequence, try doing the Love, Love, Love meditation on page 113. Concentrate on step 1, but rather than focusing on negative emotions, imagine that feelings of illness or tiredness are flowing out of your body with each exhalation.

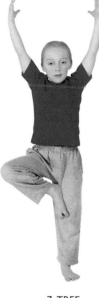

7. TREE
(page 49)

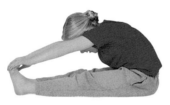

8. SITTING SANDWICH
(page 54)

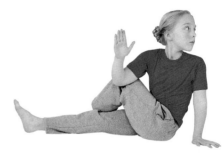

9. SAILING BOAT
(page 56)

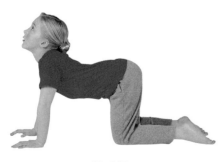

10. CAT
(page 69)

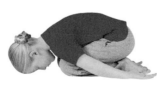

11. MOUSE
(page 68)

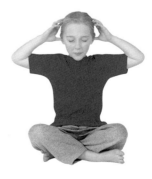

12. BEE BREATH
(page 107)

a day in the life ...

This sequence is different from the previous ones in that, here, each posture forms part of an interactive story in which you, or you and your friends or family, are the protagonists. You can make the sequence as long, short or as convoluted as you like by adding or subtracting postures or going off on tangents. Once you've got the hang of A Day in the Life ... you can make up your own stories using other yoga postures that you know. You can even fly off into outer space if you feel like it!

Lying in bed

Imagine that you are a farmer and that you are lying in bed (lie down in *Shavasana* or *Shavasana* Sandwich; see pages 32–3) after a hard day's work. As you sleep you have beautiful dreams about the fantastical lands that lie beyond the rainbow. Imagine what these lands are like – bright colours, beautiful smells, enchanting music, trees made of diamonds, and birds made of silver and gold. Visualize beautiful people, old and young, who smile at you and bring you delicious things to eat and drink. In these lands you can fly to wherever you want and all your dreams and wishes come true.

It's sunrise

Now morning is coming. Raise your arms over your head and give your body a long stretch. Squeeze your knees into your chest and rock forward and backward (Rocking Chair; see page 37). See whether you can get out of bed by rocking yourself all the way up to a standing position. The sun is just coming up over the horizon and the first rays of light are starting to warm the earth. Imagine the warm rays on your face as you do Greeting the Sun (see pages 44–5).

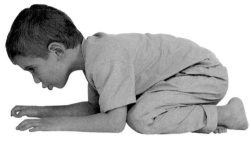

Say a silent thank you for all the goodness that the sun brings.

It's time to prepare breakfast – first you need to Sort the Rice (see page 78). Then you must Chop the Wood (see page 80) to Make a Fire (see page 68). Now slowly Stir the Pudding (see page 79) as it cooks on the fire. While you're waiting for the rice pudding, relax in *Shavasana* (see page 32) and imagine what delicious things you could add to your rice pudding. When it's ready, serve yourself a generous helping and eat it all up!

Time to go to work

Wave goodbye to your family as you set off to work. Walk like a crow (see page 88) down to the river bank. Now you have to get across to the island to feed your animals – how are you going to cross the river? You could go in your Sailing Boat (see page 56) or your Rowing Boat (see page 82); you could Build a Bridge (see pages 84–5) or you could swim (see page 93). You could even walk under the water like a Swamp Monster (see page 91).

When you get to the island, all of your animals are waiting for you to feed them. You will need a partner for this bit – one person does the animal postures (see Chapter 4 for lots of ideas) while the other person is the farmer. Then you change roles. When you are the farmer ask your animals how they are feeling today (you could get them to do Expressing Emotion on page 31). Also ask them if they have had any adventures since you last saw them. If they have, can they act them out in yoga postures?

Home time

It's getting late, so it's time for the animals to settle down. You must start making your way home while it's still light. You need to cross the river again but, if you came by boat, it has drifted away, so you'll have to Build a Bridge (see pages 44–5) or swim (see page 93) instead. You may even have to use your private Helicopter (see page 40). Now choose your favourite yoga walk (see pages 86–92) to get back to your house.

At home your friend is sitting on the porch Cradling the Baby (see page 81). You take the baby and cradle it yourself. Talk softly to it, telling it what you've been doing all day. You soon start feeling hungry so you go and make yourself a sandwich (see page 54). What will you put in it and how many will you eat?

Moon rise

Now the sun is going down and you greet the first sign of the moon in the sky by doing Half Moon (see page 51). It's almost time to go to bed, but just before you do, you must Walk the Dog (see page 86).

To get yourself ready for bedtime, lie down in *Shavasana* (see page 32) and go through all the events of the

day in your head. Try to visualize and name each of the postures that you did – see if you can remember them all in the right order. Finally, relax by doing the Sleeping Yogi (see pages 114–15) or one of the meditation exercises from Chapter 6.

The next day in the life ...

The next time you practise A Day In the Life ..., try to go on a completely different adventure or voyage. Instead of looking after animals on an island, perhaps you could feed birds in a forest (how many yoga poses involving birds and trees can you think of?) or perhaps you could go on a tour of the insect world. Let your imagination run wild!

A DAY IN THE LIFE OF AN ASTRONAUT

If you've always loved the idea of being an astronaut, try making up a yoga sequence in which you go on your own voyage into outer space. For transport, you could get into Rocket (see page 58). The first planet that you will arrive at is the moon so you could get out of Rocket and into Half Moon (see page 51). Then as you're very close to the stars you may want to make up your own yoga pose that resembles the shape of a star. When you get near to the sun you could do a few rounds of Greeting the Sun (see pages 44–5). And, of course, you're bound to meet aliens in space, so you could make up your own alien walk (and don't forget to imagine what aliens would sound like and what they would say – can you do an impression of one?). Finally, at the end of your journey you could become an inner astronaut by sitting or lying down and doing one of the meditations in Chapter 6.

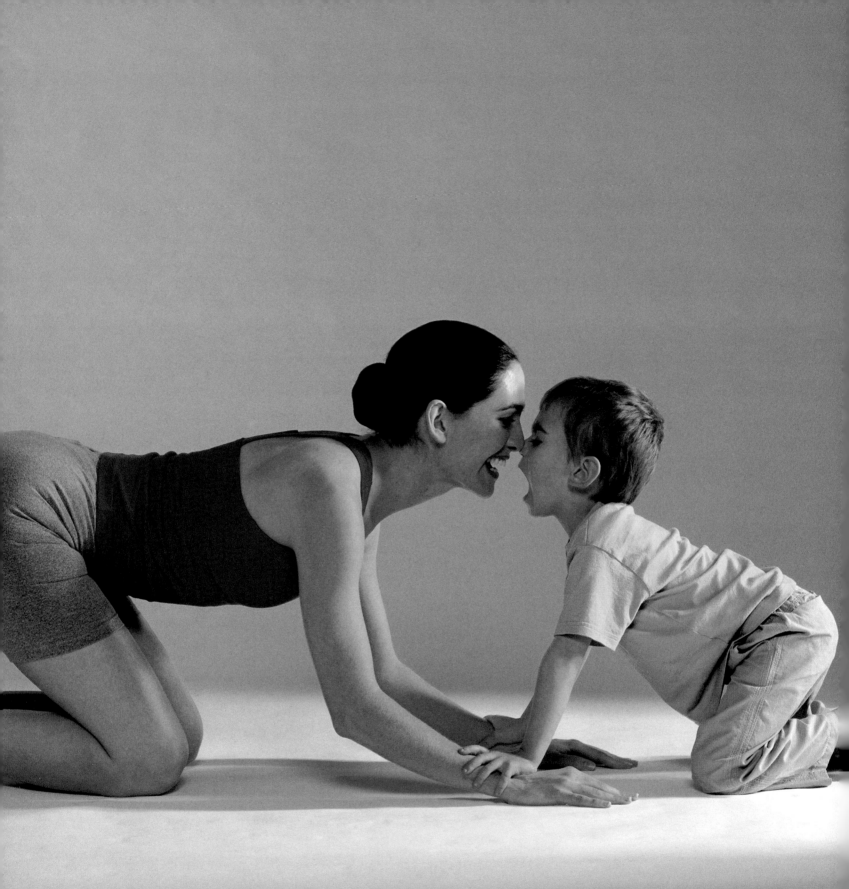

yogis at school

The aim of yoga is to help your child to blossom in every aspect of their being – physical, mental, emotional and spiritual – rather than to make them top of the class. A yoga approach to education encourages children to remain open to the wonder and wisdom of their own nature, and to work without fear of failure or craving for success. Yoga means making peace with yourself and the world around you, and meeting the challenges that life presents with skill and compassion. If your child can learn these arts, then they will have found true and lasting success, far beyond grades and certificates.

The ideas and exercises in this chapter can help your child to cope better and learn better at school. They will improve concentration and attention, and reduce the stress and anxiety that come from the pressure to perform well. And as part of an integrated yoga practice, they will have a wholly beneficial effect on your child's school life, helping them to be happier and more contented both in and out of the classroom.

learning with confidence

Building self-esteem is the first step to creating the conditions that are necessary for learning. If a child believes that they are good, intelligent and creative, they will come to embody these qualities. If, on the other hand, they are told they are bad, stupid or useless, their self-esteem will plummet and they won't be able to flourish. Psychologists at the Alice Project – an experimental learning program in India (see page 10) – found that as self-esteem increases, so do children's academic proficiency and social skills.

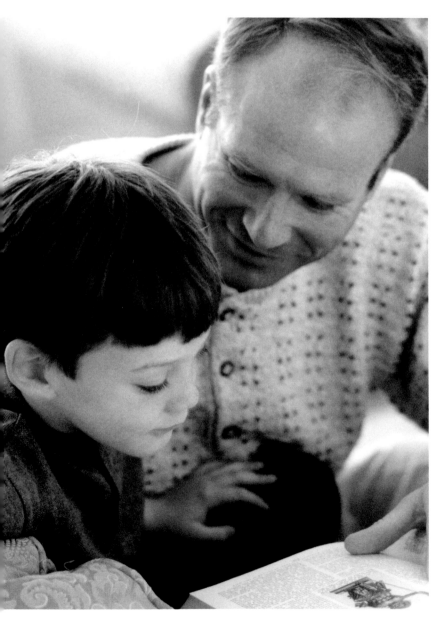

The positive and negative messages that children receive from their parents, teachers and other caregivers on a daily basis have a direct impact on their emotional wellbeing. This is why, as a parent, it's important to make positive reinforcement part of your day-to-day relationship with your child. Try to be cheerful and optimistic about events and situations in your child's life, even when things seem gloomy. Praise and encourage your child, celebrate their achievements – no matter how small – and don't hesitate to point out their strengths. This doesn't mean flattery – it just means putting the emphasis on good qualities rather than on faults.

How positive are you?

To be a truly positive influence on your child you need to think and feel positively yourself. Do you have a tendency to be self-critical? Do you compare yourself unfavourably with others? Is your outlook on life optimistic or pessimistic? Can you list five good qualities about yourself? If you think you have low self-esteem, try doing the *sankalpa* exercises on the opposite page. You will be investing in not only your own emotional health but in your child's as well.

Posture practice and meditation

Simply practising yoga on a regular basis will build self-esteem in your child. A balanced posture practice, with just the right blend of challenge and support, will teach your

Giving your child plenty of attention, encouragement and praise is the most powerful way to build up a core of self-confidence in them. Children who are self-confident are able to enjoy learning for its own sake rather than getting hung-up on success or failure.

child to move with relaxed awareness and a sense of grace. Children who do yoga tend to be self-possessed and confident in their actions and speech.

At the heart of self-esteem lies the ability to love yourself. This is an idea that can seem strange to many people. We're often socialized to believe that love is something that we direct outward – to our parents, siblings and other relatives and friends – anywhere rather than inward. It can even be easier to love our pets than to love ourselves.

Yoga, together with many other spiritual traditions, insists that to love and accept oneself is the prerequisite for transformation. Only when we believe we are worthy of love will we be able to receive the love that we need. And only when we have learned to accept love for ourselves will we be able to give it to others. This is why high self-esteem is so vitally important for the developing child. Practising meditation exercises (see pages 110–113) is a valuable way for your child to learn about and accept their innermost selves. In particular, a meditation called Love, Love, Love (see page 113) can help to cultivate feelings of loving self-acceptance. If you and your child enjoy doing this exercise, try to make it a regular part of your yoga practice or part of your child's daily bedtime routine.

Sankalpas

Another highly effective way to build self-esteem is by using affirmations, known in Sanskrit as *sankalpas*. These are positive statements of intent about who we wish to become or the qualities we wish to embody.

If children have negative ways of labelling themselves such as "I'm no good at maths" or "I'm useless at running", *sankalpas* can help them to start thinking in a new way. Some useful *sankalpas* might be "Every day I am more intelligent" or "Every day I am stronger and faster" or even "I love myself no matter what".

Work with your child to make up your own *sankalpas*. Always keep the statements positive, avoiding words such as "not" and "don't". This helps you and your child to focus on

---

THE POWER OF SELF-BELIEF

This story from the Japanese Zen tradition illustrates the importance of self-confidence. There was once a wrestler by the name of O-nami, or "Great Waves". He was immensely strong and in private nobody could defeat him. But whenever he wrestled in public he became so shy that even beginners would beat him. In desperation he went to see a great meditation master, who advised him to meditate on his own name, O-nami, and to imagine himself as huge, thundering waves sweeping away everything in their path. All night he sat and meditated on this, feeling the power grow within himself. When morning came he knew he was transformed into those mighty waves. His old self-image had been washed away, and confidence and self-esteem had taken its place. After that, nobody in the whole country could defeat O-nami. The lesson to take from this story is that anything is possible with unshakeable self-confidence.

---

the positive aspect of whatever they intend to become rather than the negative aspect that they wish to overcome. It can take time to find just the right phrase, so be ready to adapt your *sankalpa* at first. Encourage your child to keep the phrase simple and to the point and, once they have found the phrase that fits, stick with it until the *sankalpa* has done its work and they feel ready to move on to a new one.

Sankalpas can work at a very deep level of consciousness and, for this reason, it's useful to do them when your child's mind is in an open and receptive state. One of the best times to practise *sankalpas* is during a deep relaxation exercise called the Sleeping Yogi (see pages 114–15). Get your child to repeat their *sankalpa* silently three times – once before step 2 and again before step 4. Over time you will notice that this simple repetition has a huge influence on the way your child views him- or herself.

the gift of attention

If children are to learn effectively, they need the gift of attention – that quiet place of spacious, relaxed awareness where their minds and hearts are still and listening. When you see children absorbed in a game or a task, they are in this state of receptivity and it is here that true learning can take place. This is the creative space that artists know during times of inspiration. It is also the mind-space of the yogi, where relaxation and alertness coincide to create the perfect learning environment.

There are amazing stories of children trained in yoga and meditation who can memorize whole volumes of text in a staggeringly short period of time – often a matter of hours or days. This is because they are able to bring themselves at will into a state of absolute receptivity and listening. Although feats like these can seem like miracles, many of us can remember a time when we had a taste of heightened alertness and clarity – when a task seemed to be not only

The yogic approach to learning is to encourage children to be mindful – to be completely absorbed in the moment. Mindful learning means that children are able to apply their attention wholeheartedly without experiencing distraction.

effortless but blissful. One of the benefits of yoga is that it can make this state more accessible on a daily basis, to adults and children alike.

Turning off the outside world

Many children find it difficult to focus their attention for long because they are surrounded by distractions and temptations in the form of television, video games, electronic toys and computers. Add to this the fast pace of modern life, and it comes as no surprise that children have lost the ability to look inward. Being constantly "out" without ever coming back to themselves is bound to have a disastrous effect on

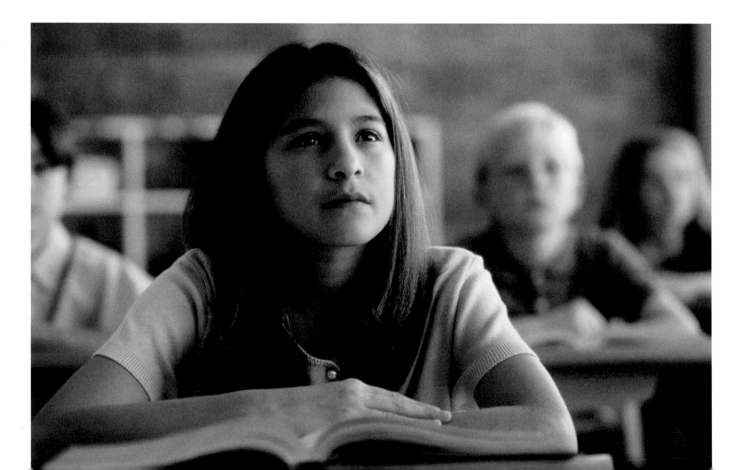

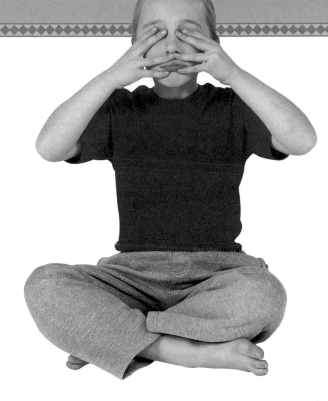

Closing the Doors is an exercise that teaches you how to gather and focus – two essential prerequisites for effective learning. By physically blocking out the sounds and images of the outside world your attention naturally comes to rest on the expansive space within you.

children's ability to manage their thoughts, emotions and behaviour, and, consequently, on their ability to learn.

To maintain a healthy mind and body, children – and adults – need a respite from the constant stimulation of modern life. They need to build a balance between their inner and outer worlds. You can help your child to do this by monitoring the degree and quality of stimulation that they are exposed to and by encouraging them to have quiet time. Sharing a regular and mindful yoga practice with your child is also one of the best ways to "turn off" the outside world.

Relax-gather-focus

To learn the art of attention you need to do three things. The first is to find the right balance between alertness and relaxation. If you are tense, you will quickly get a headache and become exhausted. If you are too relaxed, you will be scattered and unfocused. The Buddha once suggested to a musician that he be like the strings on his instrument – neither too tight nor too loose – so that the music of his meditation would be sweet. The same goes for effective learning. Yoga can bring you to the point where alertness and relaxation are perfectly balanced. So before your child starts work, do some relaxation exercises (see pages 114–15) alongside some of the concentration exercises on the following pages.

The second thing you need to do is to gather yourself. This means putting all your distractions firmly to one side, no matter how tantalizing they might be. The third thing is to focus – to bring all your attention to a single point. If you can achieve this, learning becomes effortless and enjoyable, rather than an uphill struggle.

The following exercises are designed to help your child gather and focus themselves so that attention comes easily to them. (Attention is not a skill that children are born with – it needs to be cultivated and practised.) The exercises are

largely based on the principles of *pratyahara* (gathering our mental forces into ourselves) and *dharana* (focusing our entire attention on a given object). These are the fifth and sixth limbs of yoga according to the *Yoga Sutras* (see page 18).

Closing the Doors

This exercise is about closing out the world and just sitting in silence with yourself. It allows you to return to your "listening centre" and to take a break from the noise and images with which you are constantly bombarded in your day-to-day life. Closing the Doors is a good exercise to mark the beginning of a special period of quiet time. Most children love to do the strange looking hand gesture of Closing the Doors but some find it odd – don't make your child do the exercise if they don't feel comfortable with it. Guide your child through the following instructions.

Start by finding a comfortable position such as kneeling or sitting cross-legged on the floor. Spread the fingers of both hands out (palms up), then bring your index and middle fingers together. Now take your hands up to your head and block your ears with your thumbs. Lightly place your

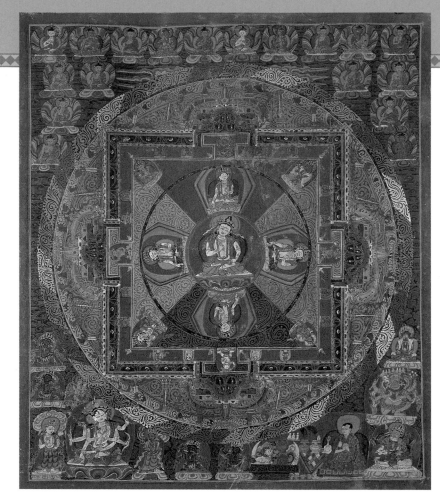

Traditionally, yogis have honed their visualization skills by visualizing mandalas such as this one. Mandalas are said to open the yogi up to the deepest truths of the soul.

You can also start to look and listen out for the pictures and the words that you have inside yourself. Imagine that you are watching a kind of internal film.

A great yogi once told the famous Indian poet-saint Mirabai to "Become so still you hear the blood flowing through your veins". By doing this she discovered herself "on the verge of entering a world inside so vast I know it is the source of all of us".

The art of visualization

One of the great secrets of learning is visualization. Fixing a picture in our mind is a skill that can be learned by most people over time. Those who have perfected it are said to have a "photographic memory".

Visualization forms part of the practices of Tantric yoga. Yogis visualize intricate and colourful geometric shapes known as *yantras* or *mandalas*. Usually made up of a circle around a centre and several "doors", *yantras* and *mandalas* symbolize the essential harmony of the universe and the infinite complexity of creation.

You can cultivate your visualization skills by practising the following exercises. As your skills improve you will find that you can apply visualization to anything that you want to learn or remember.

Drawing Inside your Mind

This exercise involves visualizing simple shapes, something which helps children to develop their visual memory. It also has a calming, focusing effect and it helps children to translate verbal instructions into non-verbal data and vice versa.

index and middle fingers over your eyes and use your ring and little fingers to press your lips together (don't do this bit if your nose is blocked). This hand position is a type of seal known as a *mudra* in yoga – it is designed to close the door of your senses. Traditionally, people practising this *mudra* would use their ring finger to narrow their nostrils to make their breath finer and slower. In this children's version, the nostrils are left open and the lips are pressed together instead as a sign of silence.

Now that you have no sights or sounds coming in and no words or noises coming out, open up your inner eyes and ears. What subtle sounds can you hear? Listen to the sound of your breathing, your heartbeat and even the singing of your blood as it rushes around your body. Do this exercise for short periods – just a few seconds at first – and talk about what you heard and felt afterward. Later on, when you get used to Closing the Doors, you can do it for longer.

NURTURING ATTENTION

The kind of attention that yoga cultivates is different from the kind of attention that was encouraged by the stereotypical Victorian schoolmaster shouting "Pay attention!" to his class. True attention is free from fear and cannot be forced. Studies by child psychologists have demonstrated that repressive and authoritarian teaching methods do not help children to learn. It's also counterproductive to make children attend to subjects that they simply aren't interested in. If your child seems indifferent to a particular area of study, think of novel ways to bring it to life. For example, in science, tell them about the latest discoveries in physics; in maths, the adventures of infinity; and in geography, the human stories behind the places and the people. Help your child to understand the relevance of what they are studying and its importance in their life.

Sit down with your child and encourage them to close their eyes and relax. Ask them to visualize a big sheet of white paper inside their head. Tell them that they are going to imagine drawing some shapes on this piece of paper. Now give your child a series of instructions about how to draw a simple *mandala*-like pattern. You'll probably need to work out your instructions in advance. Here's what you might say.

"First visualize drawing a big circle. Around the circle, and touching it, draw a square. Inside the circle, draw a triangle, with the three points touching the circle. Now, in your mind's eye, stand back and look at the pattern you have created." Remember to pause between each instruction to allow your child time to complete each stage (or give each instruction twice). Finally, ask your child to open their eyes. Give them a pen or pencil and a piece of paper and ask them to draw the shape that they have just visualized.

Vary the pattern and the shapes each time you do the exercise with your child and introduce more complexity as their visualization skills improve. You can also introduce colours. For example, your instructions could include a green circle, a red square and a blue triangle. You'll need to supply coloured pencils or crayons so that your child can try to replicate the colours when they draw the pattern on paper at the end of the exercise.

When you've finished Drawing Inside Your Mind, let your child decorate their *mandala* drawings with more shapes and colours, encouraging them to work from the centre out (in *mandalas* the centre represents the core and source of our being from which everything grows). You can use these *mandalas* to decorate the walls of your yoga space.

Another way to do this exercise is to swap roles, so that your child describes a pattern of their own design to you while you try to visualize and then draw it – this is great training in verbal communication for them and good visualization practice for you.

The Numbers Game

This game is another excellent way for children to develop their visual memory. With practice, it can enable them to memorize incredibly long lists of figures.

Sit down with your child and encourage them to close their eyes and relax. Ask them to visualize a blackboard on which they are going to write some numbers in white chalk. Start by telling them to make sure that the blackboard is clean – if it isn't, they should give it a wipe with an imaginary cloth. Now slowly read out a list of numbers to your child and ask them to visualize writing them on the imaginary blackboard.

When you come to the end of your list (start with just three numbers at first) ask your child to mentally scan the numbers and read them out backward to you. Now ask them what the first number is and then the last number. As their visual memory gets better, steadily increase the list of numbers that you read out to your child (you may find you need to write the numbers down so that you don't forget them!). Now try swapping roles so your child gets a chance to test you on your visualization skills.

Spell it Out, Spell it In

You can also apply the principle behind the Numbers Game to word spellings. Once children are familiar with the blackboard visualization technique, it can be a rapid and effective way of remembering what words look like, and it's useful if your child is having difficulty with spellings. It can even help in memorizing quotations and longer passages of text.

Follow the instructions for the Numbers Game but, instead of telling your child that they are going to write numbers on their imaginary blackboard, tell them that they are going to write a word. Now slowly spell out the letters of a word that your child would like to remember and ask them to visualize writing these letters in white chalk on the blackboard. For example, M-E-D-I-T-A-T-I-O-N. Now ask your child to spell the word back to you by visualizing it in white letters on the blackboard.

What Happened Today?

This simple visualization exercise involves looking back on the happenings of the day, something which helps children to focus on a linear series of events, and which gives a sense of coherence to their day-to-day lives. What Happened Today? is particularly good to do before bedtime because it provides a neat conclusion to the day. You can also incorporate it into the Sleeping Yogi exercise (so that it replaces the main visualization) on pages 114–15. Although it can be quite challenging at first, What Happened Today? quickly becomes a pleasure to do.

Sit down with your child and encourage them to close their eyes and relax. Explain that they are going to remember all the things that have happened to them today starting with the present moment and going all the way back through the day until they get to the point in the morning when they were still lying in bed. Ask them to visualize their day like a movie playing backward. Invite them to share with you what they see.

If you need to, you can help your child by prompting them. Remind them of the most important features of the day and encourage them to tell you what happened prior to those events. As they become more experienced at visualization they can add as much detail as they feel like.

Don't push your child to remember more than they want to during this exercise and don't worry if they get tired and give up halfway through at first – this is entirely normal. Just do whatever your child feels comfortable with. Pushing them is counterproductive because they'll be reluctant to do the exercise again.

Eagle Eyes

This exercise is an adaptation of a Hatha yoga discipline called *Tratak* which is designed to develop *dharana*, or one-pointed concentration. It is particularly good for counteracting a scattered and unfocused state of mind. Practised on a regular basis, Eagle Eyes can not only improve your child's attention span, but also make the mind quiet and ready for true meditation (see pages 108–109). The exercise is also good for the eye muscles. Guide your child through the following instructions.

Hold your left index finger up, 10 cm (4 in) in front of your nose. Stretch out your right arm at shoulder height and hold up your right index finger. As you breathe out, focus your eyes on your left fingertip in front of your nose. As you breathe in, shift your gaze to your outstretched right finger. Continue in this way for five to ten breaths, keeping your breath and the focus of your eyes soft. If you feel any discomfort in your eyes, stop immediately.

Eagle Eyes provides a good opportunity to point out one of the quirks of human eyesight to your child. They will be fascinated to find out that when they look at their left finger through first their right and then their left eye, their finger makes a sudden jump to the right. You can also try asking your child why we don't see two of everything when we have both eyes open (but be prepared to give the right answer yourself).

A slightly different way of practising Eagle Eyes is to shift your gaze from your left finger to a point on the wall or to the central point of one the *mandalas* that you made in Drawing Inside Your Mind (see pages 132–3). Alternatively, you could use a picture of a *mandala* or a *yantra* in a book. Just practise the exercise in whichever way feels most comfortable to you.

A simple variation of *Tratak* is to watch the second hand of a watch or clock for one minute with your full attention. It sounds deceptively easy. But remember that you must stay focused on the second hand without drifting off or becoming distracted for even a moment.

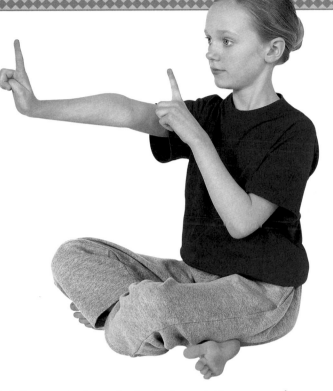

Eagle Eyes is a simple exercise that involves switching your gaze from one outstretched finger to another. Practised regularly, it teaches you to hone your attention to a single point.

THE STORY OF THE TIBETAN MONK

Once, in Tibet, a young monk was studying with his teacher, who was very strict. The teacher had to go away on business, but before he went, he gave his pupil a long and difficult passage from the sacred teachings. "Learn this by heart before I return," he said to the boy.

Nobody thought that it was possible that a boy of his age could learn such a long passage in so little time. But in spite of this, the boy spent his time playing and daydreaming. His friends and family warned him, "If you don't start learning, teacher will punish you when he gets back". But the boy played on. The days passed and the boy's family were frantic. The teacher was due back and the young monk hadn't looked at the passage.

Then, with no hurry, the boy put down his toys and picked up the book. He opened it, and read slowly through the words once. The next morning his teacher came and asked him if he had done his homework. To everyone's amazement, the boy recited the text word for word with no hesitation.

The boy went on to become one of the greatest meditation masters of the 20th century. Of course, it would be foolish to try to emulate him; according to the Tibetans, he had actually been a great teacher in a former life, and had carried over his ability to learn the teachings into this life. But the story also shows that learning happens not when we're worried about punishment or success, but when we are relaxed and focused.

exams the yoga way

Exams can be the most stressful events of a child's life. This is why it is vital, during the revision and exam period, that children practise the techniques and skills they have learned in yoga to avoid getting swept away in work and exam panic. As school life becomes more and more test-oriented from an increasingly early age, yoga has the tools to help kids survive.

Keep things in perspective

One of the most helpful ways of dealing with the anxiety of exams is to encourage your child to remember the bigger picture that is offered by yoga (see pages 22–3). When children think about their "big self" and "little self", it can help them to put exams in perspective. Suddenly, instead of being scared, children are able to approach exams in a relaxed frame of mind and with a sense of humour. Putting things in perspective not only alleviates stress, but also improves children's performance because memory works best when the mind is calm and relaxed.

Yoga can also help children to base their self-esteem on something larger and more enduring than test and exam results. As a parent you can help to reinforce this – never let your child's self-esteem be determined by how well they perform, whether it be in the exam room or on the football pitch. Once children feel sure that your love is unconditional and not dependent on their success or failure they will gain the confidence they need to grow. They will also be less anxious about exams. I strongly believe that fear of failure is never the way to assure success – this is an idea that I have reiterated throughout this book. It seems to me that fear of failure is one of the most widespread and damaging habits that we take with us into our adult lives.

During the exam period

Try to do regular yoga sessions with your child throughout the exam period. Even if they don't feel they have time, encourage them to reserve part of each day for a focused *asana* and relaxation practice. Truly relaxing breaks such as this can enhance learning and are far more productive than,

say, watching television. Your yoga sessions can be short – just 10 minutes of gentle stretching with calm, full breathing (see pages 104–5) can work wonders. If your child is feeling particularly run down or overworked, do lots of calming postures, such as gentle forward bends (see page 54). Always include one of the meditation exercises in Chapter 6 in your session.

Encourage your child to revise in the most relaxed and focused way they can. Practising some of the gathering and focusing exercises on pages 131–5 can help here. Always discourage last-minute cramming. You can help children to absorb information by reading it aloud or playing a recording of it at bedtime (or instead of step 3 of the Sleeping Yogi exercise on pages 114–15). This method works because, as we enter deep relaxation, our brain patterns change and we naturally become more receptive to information. Your child doesn't need to make any conscious effort to remember what they are hearing – they just need to allow themselves to relax. The famous Indian yoga teacher Swami Satyananda Saraswati is said to have completed the early education of his protégé using this technique.

Before an exam

Your child can benefit greatly from doing yoga prior to an exam, perhaps when they get up in the morning. Don't do anything too strenuous or stimulating. Instead, concentrate on poses that will make them feel strong and calm. A good choice would be several slow rounds of Greeting the Sun (see pages 44–5) or the Calm Me Down sequence (see pages 120–21). You can also encourage your child to do some stretches and a breathing exercise from Chapter 6

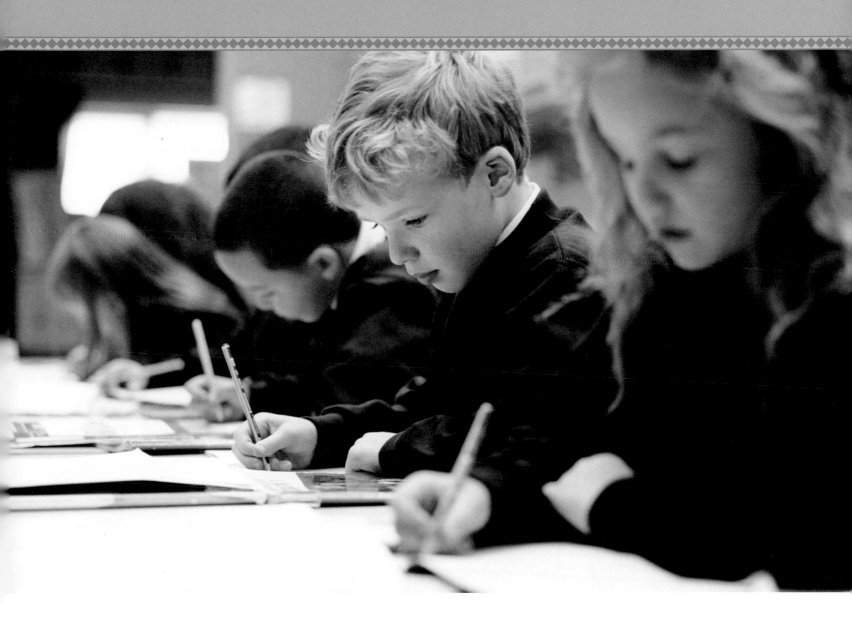

immediately before going into the exam room. Windy Tree (see page 39), Helicopter (see page 40) and the first three movements of Greeting the Sun (see pages 44–5) are ideal for waking up the spine and bringing alertness. Your child can even do some discreet stretches and twists in their chair during the exam itself.

Visualize your performance

When we are nervous we often create negative mental pictures of ourselves fumbling, panicking or losing control. Far better is to create a positive mental image, say, one in which

Children often approach exams with feelings of nervousness and anxiety. This negative mindset not only makes them feel bad, it also damages their ability to reach their true academic potential. Yoga advocates a more mindful way of approaching and tackling exams, and one which eliminates performance pressure and puts the emphasis on a relaxed approach to doing your best.

your child visualizes themselves in the exam room, writing brilliantly and with ease. This is a technique that can be applied to any difficult situation, from going to an interview to performing in a school concert. If a child believes that things will go smoothly, the chances are that they will.

conclusion

I hope this book has given you lots of ideas for practising yoga with your child, and has perhaps also inspired you to explore yoga more deeply for yourself. Ideally, you should use this book as a companion to a regular weekly yoga class with your child. You might also like to look into yoga clubs and holidays that cater for children. The internet is the first place to look around for who is teaching where. Also try enquiring at community centres and yoga schools. If there is nothing of the kind where you live, and you have a good grounding in yoga yourself, think about starting a yoga club of your own. Just a few friends in your own home once a week is a good way to begin.

I hope that in the near future, as yoga enters the mainstream, its benefits will be felt by people of all ages, through all levels of society. I hope that you can take a part, however small, in making this happen. I would especially like to see more yoga in the field of education, where it could contribute to a truly holistic approach to learning and living. It seems to me that, alongside government literacy programs, we need a curriculum for inner literacy, to teach children how to read the books of their own bodies, hearts and minds. I believe that without some kind of fundamental shift in the way that people and societies relate to the rest of the world, we risk continuing in the cycle of inequality, cynicism and despair that is threatening to destroy our planet. Yoga and meditation, taught wisely and from an early age, could provide the catalyst for this change.

So enjoy the journey of yoga with your child. Remember that the process goes on, into old age and beyond, and that, in the end, there is nowhere really to get to. As T.S. Eliot wrote:

"The end of all our exploring

Will be to arrive where we started

And know the place for the first time."

Have fun on your travels. And remember that we have at least as much to learn from children as they have to learn from us.

bibliography

Carter, F. *The Education of Little Tree* (University of New Mexico Press, New Mexico, 2001)

Eliot, T.S. *Four Quartets* (Faber and Faber, London, 1944 and Harvest Books, Pennsylvania, 1974)

Flak, M. and Coulon, J. *de Des Enfants Qui Réussissent* (Editions DDB, Paris, 1985)

Forrest, T. *I Am The Sky: Yoga for Children* (Art of Living Foundation, Santa Barbara, 2001)

Kaur Khalsa, S. *Fly Like a Butterfly: Yoga for Children* (Sterling Juvenile Books, New York, 1998)

Komitor, J.B. and Adamson, E. *The Complete Idiot's Guide to Yoga with Kids* (Alpha Books, Indianapolis, 2000)

Krishnamurthi, J. *Life Ahead* (Gollancz, London, 1963)

Luby, T. *Children's Book of Yoga* (Clear Light Publishers, Santa Fe, 1998)

Mainland, P. *A Yoga Parade of Animals, A First Fun Picture Book of Yoga* (Element Books, London, 1998)

Satyananda Saraswati, Swami *Yoga Education for Children* (Bihar School of Yoga, Bihar, India 1990)

Stewart, M. *Yoga for Children* (Vermilion, London and Fireside Books, New York, 1993)

Reps, P. *Zen Flesh, Zen Bones* (Shambhala Publications, London and Boston, 1994)

further reading

Iyengar, B.K.S. *The Tree of Yoga* (Shambhala Publications, London and Boston, 2002)
An exploration of the meaning of yoga from one of the foremost interpreters of yoga to the West.

Lazear, D. *Seven Ways of Teaching: The Artistry of Teaching with Multiple Intelligences* (IRI/Skylight Publications, Woodstock, Vermont, 1991)
A useful resource of teaching according to the individual's needs.

Liedloff, J. *The Continuum Concept* (Perseus Publishing, New York, 1986 and Arkana, London, 1989)
A fascinating and very readable anthropological study of what makes children grow up whole and happy.

Luby, T. *Yoga for Teens: How to Improve Your Fitness, Confidence, Appearance & Health & Have Fun Doing It* (Clear Light Publishers, Santa Fe, 1999)
A invaluable guide to yoga through adolescence.

Miller, John P. *The Holistic Curriculum* (Ontario Institute for Studies in Education, Canada, 1996)
A vision of a truly complete education program.

Murdoch, M. *Spinning Inward: Using Guided Imagery with Children for Learning, Creativity & Relaxation* (Shambhala Publications, London and Boston, 1988)
A goldmine of guided meditations, stories and inner journeys.

Nakagawa, Y. *Education for Awakening, An Eastern Approach to Holistic Education* (Foundations of Educational Renewal, Vermont, 2000)
Integrating approaches to learning from the Asian wisdom traditions.

Perols S. *The Human Body: A First Discovery Book* (Scholastic Books, New York and Cartwheel Books, London 1996)
A well-presented introduction to anatomy and physiology for children.

Rozman, D. *Meditating with Children* (Integral Yoga Publications, Yogaville, Virginia, 2002)
Exploring the inner life, with ideas about using meditation in education.

index

acknowledgments

Picture credits

The publisher would like to thank the following people, museums and photographic libraries for permission to reproduce their material. Every care has been taken to trace copyright holders. However, if we have omitted anyone we apologise and will, if informed, make corrections in any future edition.

Page **16** Mary Jelliffe/Hutchison Library, London; **17** Norbert Schaefer/Corbis, London; **19** Lindsay Hebberd/Corbis, London; **20** Peter Poulides/Getty Images, London; **22** Jeff Divine/Getty Images, London; **23** Campbell Mcconnell; **25** Amy Neunsinger/Getty Images, London; **27** Steve Casimiro/Getty Images, London; **108** Patricio Goycoolea/Hutchison Library, London; **111** Georgette Donwma/Getty Images, London; **112** Eastcott Momatiuk/Getty Images, London; **128** Rob Lewine/Corbis, London; **130** Rob Lewine/Corbis, London; **132** Dagli Orti/Lucien Biton Collection, Paris/Art Archive, London; **137** Mel Yates/Getty Images, London

Models

Tara and Milo Fraser, Sam Whyman, Katy Trevor-Roberts, Eleanor Sandler-Clarke, Izabella and Natasha Sanders, Sé and Cian Oba-Smith, Fenja and Kai Akinde-Hummel, Christian Denman, Jason Bailey (MOT)

Make-up artists

Lizzie Lawson,
Tinks Reding,
Nicola Coleman

Author's acknowledgments

I would like to thank the following people:

My parents, for a wonderful childhood, and continued moral support.

Marlise Meilan, for unstinting love, support and suggestions during the writing of this book, and for teaching me that everyone should be five years old at least once a day.

Valentino Giacomin, educational visionary and founder of the Alice Project, for encouragement and challenge.

Micheline Flak, one of the great pioneers of yoga education in the West, who I feel very lucky to have an association with.

Dr William Hall, physician and friend, for generous consultations on yoga and child psychology.

Nkechi Oba, children's yoga teacher, for all her help with the photos.

Sue Ray, games-master extraordinaire, who gave me my first ever yoga class, in a stable in Shropshire.

Tara and Milo Fraser, for embodying the spirit of "yoga for you and your child" throughout the making of this book.

Sheela Ziajke, for her effervescence and her ice-cubes.

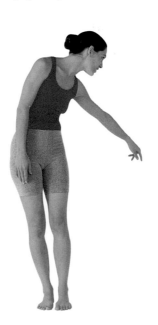
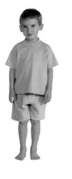